Delayed Posttraumatic Stress Disorders from Infancy

Delayed Posttraumatic Stress Disorders from Infancy

The Two Trauma Mechanism

Clancy D. McKenzie, MD

Philadelphia Psychiatric Consultation Service
Bala Cynwyd, Pennsylvania

and

Lance S. Wright, MD

Institute of Pennsylvania Hospital
Philadelphia, Pennsylvania

harwood academic publishers

Australia Canada China France Germany India Japan
Luxembourg Malaysia The Netherlands Russia Singapore
Switzerland Thailand United Kingdom

Emmaplein 5
1075 AW Amsterdam
The Netherlands

British Library Cataloguing in Publication Data

McKenzie, Clancy D.
   Delayed posttraumatic stress disorders from infancy:
   the two trauma mechanism
   1.Post-traumatic stress disorder 2.Traumatic neuroses
   3.Child psychopathology
   I.Title II.Wright, Lance S.
   616.8'521

   ISBN   90–5702–500–0   (hardcover)
           90–5702–501–9   (softcover)

Contents

Foreword

During the 65 years that I have been privileged to serve people as a psychiatrist, it has become increasingly clear that every breakthrough in the study of the human mind serves as a stepping-stone to the next level of understanding.

For nearly three decades I have followed the development of Dr. McKenzie's work in the understanding and treatment of serious emotional disorders. I have always admired his courageous tenacity in his pursuit of ideas that were beyond the boundaries of conventional psychiatry, which is where the greatest achievements invariably occur.

The two trauma mechanism represents a major contribution to the field of psychiatry. The findings reported in this book show that psychiatric illnesses are based on early trauma and follow a pattern of later activation precipitated by a major life crisis or significant stressor, and then multiple reactivation with little further provocation. This delayed posttraumatic stress disorder pattern of activation and reactivation holds true not only for schizophrenia, but also for mood disorders, anxiety disorders, psychoactive substance use disorders, eating disorders and more.

The concepts presented are based on sound psychodynamic principles supported by findings in the literature. Theory is a marriage between psychological and biological, spanning the neuroses and psychoses, from infancy to old age. It identifies mental illness as one mechanism, and psychology and biology as one process. As such, it is the beginning of a new unification theory of mental illness.

While valuable treatment concepts evolved out of the new understanding, the most powerful implications are for prevention. The early trauma that leads to emotional disorders can be identified scientifically through the research methods presented, making it possible to eliminate or modify causative factors and significantly reduce the potential for mental illness.

I believe this book is essential reading for scholars and lay persons, therapists and patients, and above all, prospective parents. I am pleased that Dr. McKenzie, together with Dr. Wright, has put this valuable work into book form for the benefit of all.

O. Spurgeon English, MD

Preface

The Mechanism

People "understand" when a car backfires next to a Vietnam veteran and suddenly he starts speaking Vietnamese, grabs a gun and hides in the woods for a few days. This is the familiar "flashback" experience: A loud noise in the present returns him to a loud noise in the distant past when his life was in extreme danger.

More terrifying than war trauma to a soldier is separation from the mother to an infant. For 150 million years of patterning of the brain, this has meant death to the mammalian infant. According to McLean (1973) to the mammalian infant, there is no more painful experience than separation from the mother. Spitz (1945) found that in some institutions, 50% of infants who were separated prior to age 2—if a good relationship with the mother had already been established and she were not replaced by another constant mother figure—simply died.

The mechanism for serious mental disorders is the same as the delayed posttraumatic stress disorder mechanism for war trauma, only instead of a loud noise precipitating the flashback decades later, it is a similar separation from some other "most important person" or group that triggers the initial return to the earlier time.

One primary difference is that the combat veteran flashes back to the mind and brain he was using at age 20, while the schizophrenic returns to the mind and brain he was using at age 1 or 2. Thus, the flashbacks of the schizophrenic reactivate not just the earlier feeling/behavior/reality/chemistry and physiology of the earlier time, but they also reactivate the earlier developmental brain structures that were active prior to age 24 months.

As the infant grows, it progresses phylogenetically from the earlier to the later developmental structures of the brain. Therefore, important neurotransmitters, involved in the schizophrenic process, increase as the flashback mechanism activates earlier parts of the brain.

The shift in brain activity away from later developmental structures results in a *disuse* atrophy of the more advanced areas of the brain—as would occur in any other part of the body which becomes inactive.

When the patient returns to a time prior to age 2 and prior to the massive development of the language centers, as in schizophrenia for example, the left posterior superior temporal gyrus atrophies proportionately more than any other region of the brain (Crow, 1990) and the patient is able to develop the language dysfunction of hearing voices.

As higher cortical thought is processed in accordance with earlier realities, aberrant neuronal pathways develop in between the corresponding brain structures, in the hippocampus. For each process taking place in the mind, a parallel process occurs in the brain itself. Careful study of the psychological mechanism and the feelings/behavior/reality of the earlier time—as compared to the changes in brain anatomy/chemistry/physiology and areas of activity—leads to the realization that biological change is the *result* of the disease process.

The Findings

Cumulative clinical observations of approximately 300 schizophrenic patients over the last 25 years have revealed a positive correlation between infant trauma in the first 18 months of life and the later development of schizophrenia. Trauma from 18 to 24 months correlates with what we refer to as "schizophrenia in the *schizoaffective range*." This refers to persons who meet the *DSM IV* criteria for schizophrenia but who exhibit a degree of warmth and have relatively fewer symptoms of schizophrenia. Most, if not all, schizoaffective patients fall into this category, along with many others suffering from the less severe forms of schizophrenia.

The same age range of origin correlates significantly with depressed subjects who have psychotic features and who may hear voices. Bipolar patients are thought to share this age of origin, but our sample of bipolar patients is too small to report this as a finding.

Trauma at age 24 months correlates with the peak incidence of asthma according to our preliminary findings, and trauma from 25 to 34 months correlates with depression that is not accompanied by voices and rarely reaches psychotic proportions.

Clinically it is possible, after very little study, to estimate with accuracy the age at the time of the original trauma—based on the behavior and the reality the patient is experiencing.

Research Confirmation

To test the validity of our cumulative observations of 300 schizophrenic patients, we surveyed patients with schizophrenia and major depression who experienced the one early trauma of birth of a sibling prior to age 36 months, and we compared the patients for sibling births between 12 to 24 months versus 24 to 36 months. Because of the importance of early trauma, and the birth-of-a-sibling trauma in particular, a high level of significance, substantially beyond the .001 level, was achieved with the first 50 subjects who had siblings less than 36 months younger.

In April 1995, Sarnoff Mednick was kind enough to test our findings on the 6,000 schizophrenic patients in the Finnish database, and he found a very high level of significance, confirming a substantially higher rate of schizophrenia among those with siblings less than two years younger. We estimate that the birth of a sibling accounts for approximately 30% of schizophrenia, and we anticipate that other infant traumas—when similarly identified and tested—will account for the other 70%.

Original Trauma

In nearly all 300 cases of schizophrenia studied, the infant trauma had one common denominator—a relative degree of physical or emotional separation from the mother as experienced by the infant. This separation is thought to produce intense pain and fear which overwhelm the infant and leave an indelible impression etched on the developing mind and brain.

Subsequent Trauma

A second important finding, gleaned from 25 years of cumulative observation, is that a trauma in the present—which is sufficiently *intense and similar* to the trauma in the past—causes the person, through a complex mental/physiological flashback mechanism, to return partially to the feelings/reality/behavior of the earlier rime. This we called the *two trauma mechanism*, and it is responsible for the commonly described "flashback" in posttraumatic stress disorders.

The trauma that precipitates the *initial* psychosis or major depression is similar to the original trauma in that it represents a separation, loss, or rejection by a "most important person" or group, whether the separation is real, imagined, anticipated, or implied. All acute stressors listed on Axis IV in the former *DSM III-R* were of this type.

People with drug and alcohol dependence had a positive correlation with a prolonged stress during infancy, and onset frequently coincided with, or was precipitated by, stress in the present.

In our view, the two trauma mechanism operates the same in all posttraumatic stress disorders of the delayed type. After the initial trauma is awakened, very little is required to reawaken or perpetuate it. With schizophrenia or depression, contact with original, nuclear family members was found to keep the earlier mind and brain active and to work against recovery. The same mechanism operates when the alcoholic takes a drink. In alcohol and drug-dependent individuals, recovery often depends on separation from original family members as well as from the abused substance.

Prevention

Our findings and theoretical constructs allow for prevention at three levels: prevention of the original trauma, prevention of a first psychotic episode in the vulnerable individual, and prevention of a relapse in persons who have an illness.

The first level of prevention is the most effective and can be accomplished through public education designed to eliminate or modify infant traumas.

The second level of prevention is prevention of an initial psychotic episode. Vulnerable individuals, i.e., those who experienced early trauma or who exhibit precursors of schizophrenia, are treated during emotional crises or at critical stages of development, to modify the impact of the second trauma in the two trauma mechanism. When this eliminates the initial flashback, the mental disorder does not occur.

The third level of prevention is prevention of a recurrence in persons who already suffer from mental illness. This is the beginning of our treatment approach.

Treatment Modalities

Correct understanding is the hallmark of treatment. Patients learn quickly the mechanisms of mental illness and the coexistence of the adult and reawakened infant minds. This provides an immediate relief, as their direction for recovery becomes clear. They strive to eliminate the infant mind and work to develop the mind of the adult. Their aim is to move out of the infant mind and brain as fast as possible, as completely as possible, and for as long as possible.

A second major principle enables the patient to accomplish his goal more quickly and completely. The patient separates from original, nuclear family because the infant is reawakened and intensified by any contact with them. This concept is illustrated with clinical examples and supported by findings in the literature.

A third major principle is the elimination of a counter transference phenomenon that dominates the relationship between patient and the entire treatment team, yet is scarcely recognized. When the patient shifts to the feelings/behavior/reality of the infant, nearly everyone relates to the patient as though he were an infant. This is counterproductive and delays or prevents a more complete recovery.

With correct understanding, a total separation from original family, and an adult-to-adult relationship with therapist and treatment team, the patient usually moves into the adult mind and brain, requires little or no medication after the first few months, and rarely suffers a relapse.

Acknowledgments

Throughout the last three decades, noted scholars and teachers have contributed valuable insights to the development and progression of the concepts presented in this text. Letters from Anna Freud, Erik Erikson, and Bruno Bettelheim added inspiration and insight, while outstanding teachers including O. Spurgeon English, Karl Menninger, Margaret Mahler, Otto Kernberg, and Victor Frankl provided the foundation for later exploration.

To be among the first to discover something new in a field that is relatively established separates one from the mainstream and invites skepticism, doubt, and even ridicule. Proof is demanded before research is funded. Dr. McKenzie cherishes the many letters of praise and endorsement from leaders in the field as the work progressed. He expresses his gratitude to the authors of those letters, including Hans Strupp of Vanderbilt, Peter Sifneos of Harvard, O. Spurgeon English of Temple, Peter Whybrow of the University of Pennsylvania, J. Martin Myers of the Institute of the Pennsylvania Hospital, and Paul MacLean, chief of brain evolution and behavior at the National Institute of Health. John deCani, chairman of the Department of Statistics at the University of Pennsylvania's Wharton Business School, was particularly helpful in endorsing the research design and statistical analysis of data. The encouragement and support from such renowned scholars as these helped Dr. McKenzie remain steadfast in his search for the cause of schizophrenia.

Appreciation is also extended to the Traumatic Stress Society and its noted scholars, including Charles Figley and Bessel van der Kolk, who peer reviewed the manuscript, and gave recognition for its contribution to the field.

Thanks also go to Bill Ingram, managing editor of the *Medical Tribune*, who was first to publicly recognize the McKenzie Method for understanding and treating serious emotional disorders, and to

Gilbert Kliman, editor-in-chief of the *Journal of Preventive Psychiatry*, for helpful suggestions and careful editing of the original manuscript. Gratitude is expressed posthumously to Bob Rodale, who nominated this work in 1986 for the Charles A. Dana Award for Pioneering Achievements in Health.

Dr. McKenzie is particularly grateful to Dr. O. Spurgeon English, teacher and mentor since 1964, who reviewed, guided, and encouraged this work throughout its development. Dr. English contributed insights and pearls of wisdom, gleaned from nearly seven decades of astute clinical observations. His open acceptance of the concepts as they developed allowed for greater freedom of thought. Without his constant feedback, this work would not have been possible.

Dr. Wright acknowledges the following individuals, who also contributed in various ways to the preparation and development of this work: Gerald H.J. Pearson, MD, pediatrician, psychoanalyst, and child development specialist; Robert Waelder, PhD, psychoanalyst, professor, and consultant; Calvin Settledge, professor of child psychiatry; Herman Belmont, MD, professor of child psychiatry; Charles Tart, PhD, states of consciousness; Stanislov Grof, MD, research in consciousness; Jean Houston, PhD, human development; Joseph Chilton Pearce, educator; Helen Devereux, educator; Glen Doman, Institute for the Achievement of Human Potential; George Devereux, anthropologist, therapeutic education; Bernard Alpeers, MD, neurologist; Lester Luborsky, PhD, research; and Robert Greenstein, MD, V.A. Clinic, PTSD, University of Pennsylvania.

About the Authors

The foundation for this clinical investigation is entrenched in psychoanalytic theory. It is a collaborative effort between two colleagues, Dr. Clancy D. McKenzie and Dr. Lance S. Wright.

Dr. McKenzie trained in adult and child psychoanalysis and psychiatry. He then devoted himself exclusively to the study of his patients, and in recent years began correlating his findings with the posttraumatic stress disorder (PTSD) literature. The clinical samples in this treatise are from his practice, and he is largely responsible for the development of psychoanalytic understanding of schizophrenia and the mathematical formulations for establishing its early traumatic origin.

Dr. McKenzie is director of the Philadelphia Psychiatric Consultation Service in Bala Cynwyd, Pennsylvania. He is the author of *Schizophrenia and the McKenzie Method*, a four-part series of audiotapes published and distributed by the American Health Association (AHA) in 1981.

Dr. Wright is a graduate of child, adolescent, and adult psychoanalytic training and has extensive experience with PTSD in veterans, substance abusers, and victims of incest and rape. He provided valuable feedback regarding conventional views and helped formulate more acceptable ways of expressing concepts to the psychiatric community at large. Dr. Wright's broad knowledge of the literature provided important collaborative findings as concepts developed, and he gathered the data for the original surveys.

Dr. Wright is an associate professor of child psychiatry at Hahnemann University in Philadelphia, and an associate professor of adult psychiatry at The University of Pennsylvania, also in Philadelphia. He has been active in many national and local professional societies, including the American Holistic Medical Association and the Philadelphia Society of Adolescent Psychiatry.

I

THEORETICAL CONSIDERATIONS

1

Literature Review

The vast majority of findings in the literature, apart from the studies of early trauma and early development, are either descriptive, or relate to predisposition, or measure what we believe are the biological results of the disease process. While description, predisposition and biological change pertain to the disease process, they are not proven causative, and exploration has not led to significant prevention. In contrast, the early traumata identified and demonstrated in this text have exceedingly high correlations with disease processes that can surface 20 to 30 years later, and these early traumata can be identified and eliminated or attenuated, making prevention possible.

Nonetheless, for completeness, we review briefly the literature pertaining to description, predisposition (genetic and in-utero viral influences), and biological change.

DESCRIPTIVE PSYCHIATRY:

Over the last century a number of descriptive scientists played an important role in the identification, description and categorization of serious mental disorders. Their work drew interest to the field and provided a framework for future study. Aside from its historical value, their work continues in the form of *DSM IV*, which is an elaboration and extension of the same efforts to categorize mental illness in a way that facilitates study, research, treatment and prevention.

Noteworthy descriptive scientists of the past include Emil Kraepelin, Eugene Bleuler, Gabriel Langfeld and Kurt Schneider. Emil Kraepelin (1856–1926), a German psychiatrist, categorized seriously disturbed individuals into three main groups: dementia praecox [schizophrenia], manic depressive psychosis, and paranoia. His main contribution to the field was his careful description and categorization of serious mental disorders.

Eugene Bleuler (1857–1939), a Swiss psychiatrist, coined the word schizophrenia, and provided the four "A"s of schizophrenia: Associations (looseness of), Autism, Affective disturbance, and Ambivalence. Gabriel Langfeld described schizophreniform psychosis, and Kurt Schneider gave us first rank and second rank Schneiderian symptoms.

From Kraepelin through *DSM IV*, classification has been largely descriptive. We believe this is because little has been understood about cause. This leaves the process of categorization in its infancy. We find it more helpful to know the age of origin of a disorder than to know that the disorder meets a certain set of diagnostic criteria, and we think that future studies likely will confirm our impression that medications and regions of brain activity are specific to age of origin—not to current diagnostic criteria.

PSYCHOLOGICAL CAUSATION:

Causation has been addressed in many ways, including psychological attempts at explanation. Sigmund Freud came the closest to the theories presented in our text when he described ego disintegration and regression as a return to a state of primary narcissism. The idea of a return to a time when the ego was not yet developed matches closely our findings. We have developed the concepts further, however, describing original trauma, precipitating trauma, the return to a specific time, age and brain site, and adding the connection between psychological mechanism and biological change.

The psychological explanation of regression, attributing it to a return to an earlier time "because" the patient was more comfortable then, is a misunderstanding of the process. While there is a tendency to adapt or "settle in" to the most comfortable aspect of the regressed state, the reason for the regression is *survival*, and in the case of schizophrenia and other serious disorders, the survival mechanism is maladaptive. Our data correlating early traumata with the later development of serious mental illness bares this out.

The most damaging of all attempts to explain the cause of schizophrenia psychologically was the attempt to blame the parent for his or her interaction with the child. The parent often suffers more than the child because of unwarranted feelings of guilt. The attempt to indite the parent was often presented in a way that was cruel and insensitive to the feelings and the needs of the parent, and this effort brought emotional destruction to lives of countless persons who already were in a state of great emotional despair.

Frieda Fromm-Reichmann (Campbell, 1989) was the first to discuss the "schizophrenogenic mother." While she and others were astute in capturing intricate nuances in the relationship, the significant mistake was to identify the unique interaction between the patient and the mother as the *cause* instead of the *result* of the disease process. Our work clearly makes this distinction: When the patient returns to the infant mind/brain/reality, *everyone* treats the patient like an infant, and this includes many mental health professionals (see chapter 16.)

Family support groups evolved as a means of self preservation, and as they grew in number and gained political influence, researchers retreated from exploration of interpersonal causes. The work of G. W. Brown (1966) had identified a strong mathematical correlation between living at home and recurrent hospitalizations, however, and this sparked a search for elements in the home environment to account for relapse. Expressed emotion in the family, referred to as the "EE" factor, was identified as the culprit, and family therapy to lower the EE factor was proven effective in reducing the relapse rate.

According to our findings, this effort does not go far enough. It is like detonating a small charge next to a combat veteran instead of a large one. The *absence* of an explosion precipitates no flashback at all. Likewise, a *zero* EE factor, brought about by a complete separation, is immeasurably better than a low EE factor.

This is not an inditement of the parent or an implication that he or she caused the disorder in any way. Even if the parent is exemplary and behaves in the most ideal way, contact can lead to relapse. The mechanism for this is the same as that between an alcoholic and the bottle. The bottle of scotch may be the finest in the world, but after the subject has "crossed the invisible line" and has become alcohol dependent, one sip returns him to the infant-on-the-bottle mind/brain/reality, and he drinks until the belly is full and passes out.

Our sympathy is with family members who often suffer more than the patient, and every effort is made to protect the parent. There may be ways in which families do share in responsibility for the perpetuation of serious disorders, however, and if so, then it is in their best interest to be aware of these factors and to learn what to do.

Two important psychological factors led to the development of family organizations: 1) strong feelings of guilt (even though unwarranted) as parents were targeted unfairly for the cause of schizophrenia, and 2) powerful psychological defense mechanisms of denial and projection, as family members could not tolerate the pain of feeling guilty. These factors influenced the direction of research for nearly two decades, and a strong desire emerged to find a biological cause or an act of God responsible. To search for the cause of schizophrenia, with the precondition that the result not precipitate feelings of guilt, is not the scientific method. Nonetheless, we have spoken with numerous mental health researchers who have said they would not dare explore possible influences related to family interactions.

Ironically, while our theories identify psychological traumata, they vindicate the parent from blame because they identify accidental traumatic experiences that happen to occur at crucial stages of development, and about which no one is aware.

BIOLOGICAL CHANGE; THE *RESULT* OF THE DISEASE PROCESS?:

All or nearly all biological change may be the result of the disease process. It stands to reason that the results of a disease process should be present in greater abundance than the cause, which would account for the large number of biological changes found in schizophrenia and other serious disorders.

Each biological finding could be molded into a separate theory of causation. Indeed some of the biological changes may influence the process itself, but in our opinion, and according to our data, the origin is associated with early emotional trauma—and biological change, for the most part, is but the result of the disease process. This includes biochemical, neuroendocrine, neuroanatomical, neurosynaptic, physiological, electrical impulse and conductivity, and change in the area of brain activity. While we do not dispute any of the biological changes that take place in schizophrenia, we find none to be causative in nature; instead, we view biological change as the result of the disease process. In our opinion, the fascination with modern technology and the discovery of the intricate biological changes are some of the main reasons for the delay in finding the cause of schizophrenia. Each new finding first has to be evaluated as to how it might cause the disorder, and many are referred to as theories even though they are not proven.

Biochemical hypotheses were updated at the *May, 1994 American Psychiatric Association Meetings* in Philadelphia: Breier presented the dopamine hypothesis, Nemeroff the neuropeptide findings, van Kammen the norepinephrine, Krystal the serotonin and Malhortra the glutamatergic findings. Our opinion remains that these are but links in the chain of reactions emanating from the return to the earlier traumatic experience.

At the same meetings, more than a dozen papers delineated changes in brain structure, including Shenton et al, Pearlson et al, Roy, De Lisi, Wyatt, Nasrallah et al, Arnold et al, Nestor et al, Shedlack et al, O'Donnell et al, Wu et al, Rossi et al, and Hokama et al. Other presentations delineated neuroanatomical areas of hypo- and hyperactivity, including papers by Russell, Gur, and Weinberger, and neuropsychological test data was presented confirming deficits in the affected areas, including papers by Andreasen et al, Nestor et al, Silverstein et al, Frecska et al, Shedlack et al, Bark et al, and Shenton et al. None proposed our theory that the individual "flashes back" to the earlier mind/brain/reality/feelings/behavior/chemistry/physiology and neuroanatomical sites in the brain that were active at the time of the first trauma during infancy. Our theory explains the hypoactivity and the resultant *disuse* atrophy of the phylogenetically more advanced structures of the brain, and it explains the increased activity of the phylogenetically older structures as well. In 1941 Kardner coined the term "physioneurosis" to describe the cellular, physiological "remembering" that accompanied what is now known as the "flashback." When the flashback is to a time prior to the development of the more advanced structures of the brain, the individual begins using the earlier structures to the exclusion of the later developmental structures, and the result is a *disuse atrophy* of the more developed portions of the brain.

PREDISPOSITION: GENETIC AND IN UTERO VIRAL AND NUTRITIONAL INFLUENCES:

Present genetic data must be reexamined and scrutinized in terms of the new insights and understanding of the relationship between trauma in the first two years of life and the later development of schizophrenia. Surveys from the 1930s reveal that siblings of a schizophrenia proband have an 8% chance of developing the disorder, and dizygotic twins (DZTs) have a 12% chance. **Genetically, however, DZTs are the same as non twin siblings** (Kaplan and Sadock, 1994.) *Therefore, if the 8% figure is accurate for the non twin siblings, then the additional 4% for DZTs cannot be attributed to genetic factors.*

Furthermore, using the trauma hypothesis, the additional four are the result of a trauma at an age of vulnerability for the development of schizophrenia, and the trauma was sufficient to result in the later development of schizophrenia in the four individuals. These four have siblings who are the same age and who had the same age-specific vulnerability at the time of the trauma. Thus the trauma that caused schizophrenia in each of them likely caused the schizophrenia in their twins.

Since 8 of the 8 non-twin siblings (NTSs) were not the same age, they did not suffer the same trauma at the same age. One could have been 11 or 12 months old and the other 22 or 23 months old at the time of the same trauma, placing both at risk for schizophrenia, but at least they were not affected at the same age by the same traumatic occurrence. They still can be affected by the same *type* of trauma at the same age, however, in instances of poor parenting, or sickly or periodically depressed or addicted or periodically absent parents who are traumatic to all children of a particular, vulnerable age. This could account for any or all of the 8 NTSs who develop the disorder.

According to Robert Cancro (1993), 90% of schizophrenics do not have a family history of schizophrenia. In the overall population, slightly more than 1% have schizophrenia, and the vast majority of these do not have a schizophrenic first degree relative. Therefore we must subtract one more from the non-twin siblings and from the remaining percentage of dizygotic twins who might have schizophrenia on a genetic basis alone. This leaves still fewer NTSs and DZTs who might have schizophrenia strictly on the basis of genetics.

Based on our findings, all may relate to early traumata, and we seriously question whether a person can flash back to infancy without having experienced an original trauma then. *Even if early traumata are necessary for the later development of all serious disorders, however, this does not preclude a genetic predisposition in an undetermined number of cases.* We have no attachment to any particular result from this exploratory process, but we think that the relative degree of importance of a genetic predisposition has yet to be determined. Early trauma, however, appears necessary for schizophrenia to occur.

SECOND TRIMESTER FACTORS:

According to Mednick (1987, 1988) and Barr & Mednick et al (1990), there is a significant increase in schizophrenia among those whose mothers were subjected to influenza epidemics during the sixth month of gestation. Butler et al (1994) and Lyon and Bracha (1994) found nutritional factors and Brown et al (1994) found famine in the second trimester of pregnancy to correlate with an increased risk for schizophrenia. Huttunen and Niskanen (1978) found that the loss of the father of the fetus in the second trimester correlated with an increased risk for schizophrenia in the offspring.

Mednick (1987), Dykes & Mednick (1992), and Cannon & Mednick (1993) reported detailed studies that distinguished between etiological factors including viral influences in the sixth month of pregnancy, obstetrical and birth trauma, separation in the first five years of life, increased ventricle brain ratios (VBRs), autonomic sensitivity, and genetic factors. The work appears carefully conducted and well thought out, particularly in the 1987 article. Each time a factor is attributed to genetic loading, however, we are able to attribute it to trauma in the first 24 months of life as well:

1. In the 1987 article Mednick places early maternal separation at the top of the list of characteristics distinguishing the sick from the well and the control groups, and he identifies the high risk (HR) children as being more reactive on skin conductance measures, but separation from the mother during infancy produces an immediate drop in skin temperature (Mizukamia, 1987), and early trauma leads to delayed type post-traumatic stress disorder from infancy, which leads to autonomic instability.

2. Any second trimester threat such as viral, chemical, famine/nutritional, paternal loss, or maternal crisis, and any complication of pregnancy and birth, incubation, hospitalization or operative procedures including circumcision, may serve as an *antecedent trauma*, and antecedent traumas are known to predispose to increased severity of subsequent traumas—which would include the other traumas during infancy that correlate with the later development of serious mental disorders.

3. Early onset schizophrenia in the mother correlates with increased severity of her schizophrenia, and a more severe schizophrenia in the mother correlates with more emotional distancing and physical separations from the infant for reasons of the mother's hospitalizations.

4. Fixing on the early trauma—in utero or in the first 24 months of life—or especially the later flashbacks to the earlier trauma, activates the phylogenically earlier structures of the brain to the partial exclusion of the more advanced regions, accounting for a

disuse atrophy of higher structures, an increased activity in the earlier regions containing more of the critical neurotransmitters, and the development of aberrant neuronal pathways in between.

5. The correlation between the ventricle/brain ratio (VBR) and paternal spectrum illness is understandable because a mentally ill father can upset a household and thereby affect the mother-infant relationship. Thus the father's influence can be his contribution to the trauma of early separation from the mother instead of his addition to the genetic load. The brain atrophy is related to the shift of brain activity to the primitive regions that were active at the time of the early trauma.

We have not closed the door on the genetic factor; we are just noting that we can explain all the changes on the basis of early trauma alone. More research is needed to establish preponderance. **To this end we hope someone will evaluate the incidence of schizophrenia in the offspring of healthy MZTs who are discordant for schizophrenia, because *genetically* they are identical to the ones with schizophrenia, and therefore genetically—if everything relates to genetics—there should be a 12% and a 40% chance for schizophrenia, depending on whether one or both parents are healthy MZTs discordant for schizophrenia.** This would *help* sort out genetic load versus familial trauma, although some familial factors apart from obvious trauma still may carry forward.

Crow and Done (1992) studied 16,268 women exposed to the 1957 influenza epidemic during pregnancy and did not find an increased incidence of schizophrenia in their offspring. Crow (1983) also speculated about a possible viral etiology after birth to account for such things as seasonal variation and an increased incidence among apartment dwellers, but Kaufman et al (1988), after injecting primates and guinea pigs with brain tissue from schizophrenic patients, found no behavioral or neuroanatomical pathology. We believe the same findings can be explained better by early trauma. Mothers may have seasonal affective disorders at a peak age of vulnerability for schizophrenia in the infants' first two years of life, and persons dwelling in close quarters may be more stressed and prone to rejecting.

Another interesting study might be to identify the incidence of schizophrenia among those who were 12 to 24 months old during the first month of the 1929 stock market crash—versus those who were 12 to 24 months old the same month two years prior to the crash.

CONCORDANCE:

According to Nelson (1993) and Schwartz (1988), 47% of MZTs of a schizophrenic proband develop schizophrenia, as opposed to 12% of DZTs. Cancro (1993) points out that the concordance would be closer to 30% instead of 47% in MZTs if one were to include twins in whom both carry the gene but neither express it. According to present data, if the gene is present (assuming this factor is a gene), there is a 49.82% chance of expression in one or the other of the two, a 22.09% chance of expression in both, and a 28.09% chance of expression in neither. Regardless how concordance is calculated, the occurrence in MZTs is appreciably greater than in DZTs. This is a powerful argument against a *predominant* viral or nutritional etiology, since both twins live in the same fetal environment and receive similar nutrition.

If the primary cause of schizophrenia were viral, nutritional, or paternal loss factors in the second trimester of pregnancy, we would expect one percent instead of eight percent non-twin siblings to have the disorder, and we would expect the percentage of DZT and MZTs of schizophrenia probands to be equal instead of 12% of 47% respectively. *Therefore we can rule out a substantial viral, nutritional or paternal loss influence in the second trimester of pregnancy because MZTs and DZTs are exposed to the same environmental influences and should have the same chance of infection, famine/mal-nutrition and paternal loss*, not a 4 to 1 ratio of MZTs over DZTs.

In deference to the extensive research pertaining to second trimester etiologies, we note the infrequency of twins (about 1.5% in the overall population). The influence of a virus or a famine can still be identified in time-limited epidemics, while the difference in concordance between MZTs and DZTs remains, corresponding to the vast majority of calendar days/years. Viral/nutritional influences still could not be the primary cause of schizophrenia, however, because of the similarity in environment of twins, and the far greater concordance among MZTs as opposed to DZTs.

What factors other than genetic can account for the increase in concordance for schizophrenia among MZTs over DZTs? Back to the two trauma theory:

DZTs can differ medically. One might have a cleft palate and separate from the mother for hospitalization and operative procedures. Many other congenital malformations can require separation for medical attention, and there may be increased susceptibility to infection in one DZT over the other. In DTZs one may be more prone to rheumatic fever than the other, or to asthma or allergies. Thus with

DZTs there is a greater chance of one being separated (and therefore traumatized) for medical reasons, whereas with MZTs when one is traumatized for medical reasons the other is more likely to be traumatized at the same time (age).

MZTs are also treated more alike than DZTs. With DZTs there is a greater chance of one being rejected more than the other, for transference reasons on the part of the parent, or because of **temperament** on the part of the child, causing one twin to be more agreeable and enjoyable than the other. Either factor causes one to experience early trauma that the other does not. One DZT may be teased, punished, neglected or criticized at a crucial, vulnerable stage of development. This too can account for less concordance among DZTs than among MZTs.

Thus, because of medical differences in dizygotic pairs, it is more likely that DZTs will be discordant and MZTs will be concordant for traumatic separations, and because of psychological factors of transference on the part of the parent and *temperament* on the part of the infant, it is more likely that DZTs will be discordant and MZTs will be concordant for the trauma of emotional separation during crucial stages of development.

At the other end of the spectrum, when a schizophrenic reaction is precipitated later in life by a "similar" trauma in one twin (either MZT or DZT), the shift to the earlier mind/ brain/reality causes the parents and everyone else to relate to the patient in a parent-infant transference. An interesting finding by Gordon (1987) supports our observation of the sudden shift in the transference relationship of the parent: Mothers of adult children who suddenly became quadriplegic, responded in a transference psychotic way, relating to the offspring as they did initially when the infant could not walk or even feed itself. They would darken the room, insist everyone be quiet, and eat the patient's food—claiming they fed him. This dates back to breast feeding or in utero when the mother eats a meal and quips "I just fed the baby." This is a powerful mechanism and probably applies when the adult child reverts to the infant mind in schizophrenia. It is conceivable that this pathological transference might be transferred again onto a MZT more often than onto a DZT, and onto a DZT more often than onto a non-twin sib. Relating to the healthy twin in a pathological parent-infant transference might then have a schizophrenogenic effect (if we dare to use that word.) We do not regard this as a primary mechanism, but in the rare instance of MZTs concordant for schizophrenia, this must be studied and considered as a possibility for the second twin who develops schizophrenia.

One does not arrive at new ideas without considering new possibilities. All possibilities must be considered equally: This is the scientific method. At the risk of credibility, let us explore a topic that can be found in the literature only at the end of Cluster "A" in *DSM IV*, i.e., let us consider thought transference. Anna Freud (personal correspondence, 1973) expressed great interest in findings related to thought transference in children, and she was very open to exploration of the subject matter. While 60% to 80% of the general population reports having experienced such phenomena, only one article in the literature dared refer to it—according to Anna Freud—and this was an article by Dorothy Burlingham which first appeared in German in 1935. If Anna Freud was open enough to explore the possibility, maybe we can too.

Considering the extraordinary examples of monozygotic twins reared apart not knowing of one another's existence, yet sharing identical interests, clothing, hobbies, and professions, it seems incredible to believe that each picks out a wife with the same name, works for a fire company of the same name in a different part of the country, and sports the same mustache—all as a result of genetics. This thought is at least as incredible as the possibility of thought transference. With MZTs reared apart, there are phenomena occurring which defy explanation, and which have not been explored. We must not make assumptions without putting them to the test. Persons who study thought transference consider likeness an important factor. They sit in the same position and synchronize their breathing with the subject, for example. How much more alike can a person be than to share identical cells? This must be explored and can be explored. Conceivably this could account for a portion of concordance, whether the twins are reared together or apart.

MZTS REARED SEPARATELY:

Monozygotic twins reared by adoptive parents have the same rate of schizophrenia as their twins reared by their biological parents (Kaplan and Sadock, 1994). On the surface this would seem to suggest that genetic influences outweigh familial ones. Many factors need closer scrutiny, however. The child who is adopted out may experience a traumatic separation from biological parents, and depending on the age this occurs, the separation may cause the disorder. The parent who adopts out one of a MZT pair *during the age of greatest vulnerability* is not in touch with the feelings and needs of the infant and thus has a pathological distance in the relationship. Therefore both the adopted out and the twin who stays with the biological parents may be subjected to special traumata at a vulnerable age. They may both undergo physical separations at the same early age because of congenital malformations that result in separations for hospital procedures. Studies related to siblings reared in different homes may draw erroneous conclusions if the studies do not take into account the trauma of early separation and do not distinguish the exact age at time of separation. Early trauma of separation may be the most important variable there is, and if the existence of an important variable is not accounted for, the results may be misinterpreted.

BIPOLAR DISORDERS:

Genetic factors are considered even more important in bipolar disorder, and according to Kaplan and Sadock (1994) 50% have at least one parent with depression— but psychodynamically the origin of bipolar disorder is a mother who is periodically depressed! The concordance for MZTs is 67% and concordance for DZTs is 20%—but the same arguments that apply to twins of schizophrenia probands may apply to twins of bipolar probands.

ADOPTION:

There has been further question as to whether or not adoption increases risk. Adoption significantly increases risk of mental illnesses in adopted children, according to the *data* presented by Zill (1985). The most important factor for the development of a specific disorder is the age at the time of the separation. This has been terribly misunderstood. For example, Breier et al (1988) conducted an excellent, comprehensive investigation to determine the effects of loss of a parent on a child, but the 90 subjects studied varied in age at time of loss from 2 years to 17 years! Our findings indicate that the psychoses relate to trauma prior to 24 months, and the non psychotic major depressions appear limited to trauma occurring between 25 and 35 months. We search for differences in subjects who were traumatized at ages one month apart, over the course of the first 36 months of life, and at two or three months apart the differences can be dramatic.

PARENTS OF SCHIZOPHRENIC PATIENT:

A child with one schizophrenic parent has a 12% prevalence for schizophrenia, while a child with two schizophrenic parents has a 40% prevalence for the disorder. The rate of hospitalization alone, for the schizophrenic parent, would account for a sharp increase in traumatic separations, and the emotional separation produced by having a schizophrenic parent would also account for an increase in the disorder. Even a mother's failure to touch the infant has been shown to lead to failure-to-thrive (Polan & Ward, 1994.) **Until these phenomena are studied, we cannot draw conclusions regarding genetics and the increased prevalence of schizophrenia among those who have schizophrenic parents.**

DERMATOGLYPHIC ASYMMETRY:

Fluctuating Dermatoglyphic Asymmetry (FDA) (as measured by fingerprint asymmetry) is used as a proposed marker for second trimester cell migration, and has been associated with schizophrenia and homozygosity at HLA Class II antigens (HLA DR and HLA DQ antigens.) "The resultant maternal-fetal HLA compatibility has been associated with poor fetal outcome, and theoretically may be a genetic vulnerability factor for schizophrenia" (Perkins and Gilmore, 1994). We like this kind of study because it appears to eliminate the familial or early trauma variable. Thus far there is insufficient data to be significant, but the work is promising and needs to be continued.

CRANIOFACIAL ANOMALIES:

Schizophrenic patients displayed significantly more facial anomalies than controls, and the facial anomalies were attributed to genetic and/or environmental factors between the 8th and 22nd week of gestation, suggesting this period may be critical to the etiology of schizophrenia (Lane et al,1994.)

This brings to mind the fetal alcohol syndrome with its facial anomalies, mental retardation and attention deficit/hyperactivity disorders. While the facial anomalies logically can be attributed to the effects of alcohol in utero, the developmental problems including retardation and attention deficit/hyperactivity disorder can also be related to having a mother who is periodically intoxicated, institutionalized or emotionally/mentally otherwise unavailable to provide the important stimulation needed by the developing infant.

Thus, with craniofacial anomalies we may think we are studying a correlation between schizophrenia and craniofacial anomalies, while we really might be studying a substance dependent mother who because of her dependence causes a chemical trauma in utero, producing the physical anomalies, and an emotional trauma during infancy producing the schizophrenia. This must be closely scrutinized. Such a factor could also be a possibility in dermatoglyphic asymmetry.

EYE MOVEMENT:

According to Holtzman (1994), Spatial working memory capacity of the prefrontal cortex is impaired in many schizophrenic patients and in about 40% of their first-degree relatives. The relationship between the deficits and the abnormal smooth pursuit eye movements is highly significant, suggesting a shared brain mechanism for the two functions and possibly a relationship with schizophrenia. Positron emission tomography demonstrates the area of brain activity during the eye movements, which suggests neuro- anatomical loci for brain dysfunction in schizophrenia.

Once more, as with the atrophy of the left posterior superior temporal gyrus, we attribute this to the *result* of the disease process—i.e., a *disuse* atrophy that occurs when the individual shifts or flashes back to the mind and brain he was using prior to the development of the left posterior superior temporal gyrus and prior to the full development of the smooth pursuit eye movement centers in the prefrontal cortex. When shifting to the earlier time, a time prior to the development of the particular function and brain center, that particular region of the brain becomes inactive, resulting in *disuse* atrophy and loss of function.

The impaired working memory capacity in 40% of first-degree relatives is interesting and calls for further exploration. According to Cancro (1993), 90% of schizophrenia has no family history. Thus the 40% could be factors other than genetic. It is possible that the testing for the impaired memory capacity is sensitive and measures a subclinical disorder in first degree relatives. Conceivably, traumatized parents might be more likely to traumatize their own offspring. A reciprocal phenomenon may also occur: Parents who relate to the patient in a parent-infant transference, sometimes seem to resonate with the phylogenetically earlier structures of their child's brain, developing secondary traits of schizophrenia and becoming rigid and inflexible themselves. It is as though to communicate better they must make a subtle shift to the same earlier region of the brain. While this concept may be new, it is not entirely new. A chameleon effect is recognized in other clinical situations. A depressed person can impact on another individual, and the anxiety of an anxious person can be contagious and transfer onto others. The hyperactivity of a bipolar in a manic state can carry over to the examiner, and a person in a state of deep relaxation has a calming effect on others. Persons engaged in conversation assume the same body posture. This is a natural tendency in communicating. Two persons playing a piano duet are relating through their premotor cortices. Thus a subtle shift to the same region of brain activity is but an extension of a process we already recognize. The scientific method is to explore all possibilities, and that is why we go beyond what we have proven to suggest areas of investigation that are speculative at this time.

CHROMOSOMES:

According to Kaplan and Sadock (1994), more than half of the chromosomes have been associated with schizophrenia in various studies, and the most commonly reported are the long arms of chromosomes 5,11,18, the short arm of 19 and the X chromosomes. At best, the literature indicates a possible heterogeneous genetic basis for schizophrenia, and none would compare the genetic findings to those found in neurological disorders. With mental illness the words "dominant" or even "Mendelian recessive" are never heard; instead the descriptions are couched in terms such as "phenotypic variant of a genotypic disorder" or "polygenic with incomplete penetrance."

DSM IV provides a reasonable note of caution that "Although much evidence suggests the importance of genetic factors in the etiology of schizophrenia, the existence of a substantial discordance rate in monozygotic twins also indicates the importance of environmental factors." The DSM is not able to identify the environmental factors, however. From our text it should be evident that the environmental factors are predominantly traumata occurring in the first two years of life. While we have conducted only a small portion of the research needed, we have provided a simple means of determining mathematically the importance of each trauma at each age during infancy.

Often there is too little distinction made in the literature between familial and hereditary, and there is a tendency to try to force everything into a genetic model. It is obvious that there are genetic factors. Anyone who can see there are tall people and short people, weak and strong, must surmise that genetically there are weak and strong minds as well. We are unable to draw any conclusions about genetic studies at the present time, however, other than they need to be re-evaluated in light of the additional variables we have presented.

SUMMARY OF LITERATURE REVIEW:

In the history of the exploration of serious mental disorders, early scientists contributed by identifying, describing, and organizing them into categories, an effort that continues today with *DSM IV*. Freud described a returning to a stage of development prior to ego development. Many unsuccessful attempts were made to simply blame the parents as causing the disorders. Biological research uncovered amazing findings related to the chemistry, physiology, neuroendocrinology, neurosynaptic transmission, conductivity, areas of activity and neuroanatomical changes that coexist with the disorders—but these remarkable findings relate largely to the results of the schizophrenic process and therefore cannot contribute meaningfully to primary prevention. The great interest in biological findings, coupled with the influx of funds to find new biological treatments, may have served to delay the discovery of the importance of early traumatic origin. This does not detract from the value of the biological efforts, because treatment can occur at any level—just as a chain can be broken at any link.

There are factors that *cause* the illness, factors that *predispose* to the illness, and factors that are the *result* of the illness:

1. The factors that are the result of the illness are present in greatest abundance, because when one has the illness there are changes in family relationships and there are countless biological changes that also take place as a result. This is a one to one ratio. If a person has the illness he has biological changes that go along with it, and family relationships necessarily change.

2. The factors that contribute to the illness include genetic strengths and weaknesses, antecedent trauma including viral, chemical (substances), emotional, nutritional and obstretical influences before birth, birth trauma, and other stresses that intensify the experience of the critical early trauma when it occurs. Contributing stressors also are present later in life and serve to augment the

traumatic experience that precipitates the first acute "flash-back"/illness.

3. The factors viewed as causative in nature are the early traumata. Persons with serious mental disorders have early traumata at ages that can be estimated clinically, and the age of the trauma can be confirmed as long as the history is known. Likewise when a severe early trauma is identified, usually the feelings, reality and behavior of the patient match the stage of development at the age the traumatic event occurred. Research surveys confirm these findings.

The trauma from infancy has one common denominator, a threat of separation from the mother as experienced by the infant. The precipitating factor later in life that causes the acute onset of the *initial* illness is always a "similar" separation, rejection or failure that triggers a flashback to the earlier experienced threat of separation, which then overwhelms the individual.

Our findings do not conflict with biological findings, nor do they conflict with viral or hereditary predispositions—but our findings do indicate a one to one correlation between serious mental disorders and traumata at specific ages for each disorder. Without the early trauma there is not the early trauma site and the early gestault to which to return, and there cannot be the specificity between the age of the original trauma and the symptoms exhibited by the patient.

2

Historical Considerations, Method of Investigation, Early Trauma, and the Two Trauma Mechanism

BASIS FOR CLINICAL INVESTIGATION:

Sigmund Freud (1894) had attributed the causes of the neuroses to trauma during childhood and later to fantasies that developed during childhood. Bruno Bettelheim (1967, 1969) attributed infantile autism to trauma during the first 18 months of life, and Margaret Mahler (1955, 1968, 1979) attributed the cause of certain childhood psychoses to pathogenic experiences in the first 18 months of life,—but there was a gap in psychoanalytic understanding regarding the cause of adult forms of schizophrenia.

Harlow (1958, 1965, 1971, 1979) demonstrated the profound effect on primates of being reared by a terry-cloth mother. Spitz (1945, 1975) showed that 50 percent of human infants suddenly deprived of a mother, after having been raised exclusively by that mother, died of anaclitic depression by age two. Anna Freud (1953, 1954, 1960, 1963) furthered these findings and found that a single, uninterrupted mother figure, instead of a continual rotation of caregivers, eliminated the anaclitic deaths.

Thus, the first author suspected infant trauma in the development of adult forms of schizophrenia, and in particular he suspected trau-

21

ma related to separation from the mother. He therefore began to take careful note of the early histories of all patients, with particular attention to events that might have been experienced as traumatic by the infant.

METHOD OF INVESTIGATION:

One particular trauma proved more useful to log than all others because it provided the age of the patient when it occurred. This was the birth of a sibling. Even in the elderly, it usually could be determined immediately how many months old the patient was when the original trauma occurred. The birth of a sibling also proved useful for another reason: It was found to be highly traumatic to many infants.

After years of cumulative observations on approximately 300 schizophrenic patients, certain characteristics began to correlate with the birth of a sibling trauma at specific early months. This then allowed for inferences as to when other patients without siblings had been traumatized, and ultimately led to the identification of other traumas.

If ten patients experienced the world in a similar bizarre way, and if each of the ten had a sibling born at age 16 months, then the next time a patient was found to experience the world in the *same* unusual bizarre way, it could be hypothesized that *something* happened to that patient at age 16 months as well. Careful evaluation of case histories regularly revealed that something caused the infant to be terrified of separation from the mother at the age in question. Approximately one chance in three it was the birth of a sibling, and two chances in three it was one of the many other early infant traumas which similarly caused the infant to feel threatened with separation from the mother.

Mahler (1979) noted the profound impact of the birth of a sibling on the older child. She did this through direct observation and prospective study. We arrived at the same findings through cumulative retrospective analyses, and confirmed the findings statistically through patient surveys.

Upon discovery of the newborn, the older child frequently fears being displaced and may be terrified of abandonment and death—or may be overwhelmed by feelings of sadness, loss and grief. The fear of separation is probably the greatest fear in infancy and early childhood. Children who are dying from cancer fear separation more than pain or death (Kaplan & Saddock). Paul MacLean (1983) described early separation as the most painful experience to all mammalian species. It elicits the cry response, which is a desperate attempt to bring the mother back. The pain and fear and the cry response associated with separation have been built in through natural selection over the course of 120 million years of evolution of the old and the new mammalian brain. In mammalian species, separation from the mother is tantamount to death, which is why it is such a painful and terrifying trauma to many infants.

Anaclitic depression has been studied in both human and animal populations (Spitz, 1945; Harlow 1958, 1965, 1979; Bettelheim, 1967; Freud, A., 1953, 1954, 1963; Freud, A. and Bowlby, 1960), and it is so overwhelming, painful and frightening that it frequently results in marasmus and death. Couple this with the fact that many studies indicate the younger the creature is, the more it is affected by trauma (See comparisons with adult trauma in Chapter 5).

Thus, the birth of a sibling can be extremely traumatic to many infants. The first child may have the mother all to itself for a period of time, and it is totally dependent on the mother. When the mother is absent for a few days, the child may be frightened. When the mother "finally" returns, holding and feeding a new baby, the first child may be far more traumatized than most realize. *This is not a matter of sibling rivalry;* the retrospective clinical projections locate the damaged developmental stage as being specific to the age at birth of the next sibling and identify the trauma as being experienced as extremely intense and life threatening. Thus, the first child may be terrified that it has been displaced. If the child then is sent off to the grandmother's house, the initial trauma is in place. The potential exists for a later "flashback" to this earlier mind/brain/reality, should a "similar" trauma occur later in life.

The precipitating trauma later in life is similar to the original trauma in that it is usually a separation or rejection from an important person or group, whether it is real, imagined, anticipated, or implied. From cumulative observations, as well as patient surveys combined with natality statistics (U.S. Dept. of Health and Human Services, 1988), the authors found a much greater than expected incidence of schizophrenia among those who have a sibling born in the first 24 months of life. By conservative calculation, the risk of developing schizophrenia is greater than one chance in 18. Large scale studies are needed with well defined comparison groups to determine more precise levels of risk and age of origin for each specific disorder and each specific symptom.

Thus, the selection of the one trauma for study, i.e., the birth of a sibling, proved fortuitous in two ways: first, it provided an immediate documentation of age at which the trauma occurred, and second, it represented an extremely upsetting and terrifying experience to many infants.

IDENTIFYING OTHER EARLY TRAUMATA:

After symptoms were correlated with specific agesof origin, using the age at the birth of a sibling parameter, it became possible to identify other early traumas. For example, one schizophrenic patient broke into an apartment and ate all the ice cream. Clinically, his behavior and reality matched that of others who had siblings born at age 18 months. The history therefore was searched for what else might have occurred at that time. The father then revealed that on New Year's Eve, when the child was *exactly* 18 months old, his wife caught him having an affair, which produced a major crisis in the family and caused her to plan to leave him. Regardless how much a mother may love her child, if a crisis such as this occurs and totally devastates and disrupts her thoughts and feelings, she suddenly becomes *emotionally absent* to the child. This example therefore identifies another early trauma in addition to the birth of a sibling; i.e., if the mother suddenly becomes terribly upset and distracted, the infant can become frightened as he quickly senses that he has lost her attention and devotion. Had the authors not known clinically that the trauma was from age 18 months, the trauma would have been more difficult to identify. Using this means to help locate other initial trauma over the course of 25 years, the authors found that nearly all trauma to the infant has *one* common denominator: the infant feels threatened by a relative degree of physical or emotional separation from the mother.

Another schizophrenic patient, a healthy 21 year old man, was convinced he would never walk again because his feet hurt. His reality resembled the reality of other schizophrenics traumatized at age 12 months, and his *primary symptom* also identified the reality "everyone else can walk, but I cannot," which is most intense just prior to walking. Based on the clinical evaluation, and on the fact that there were no younger siblings, the family was asked if something caused the mother to be very upset at that time. History then revealed the patient had a brother who died when the patient was 12 months old. While the patient presumably was not attached to the brother, the mother certainly was, and she became terribly distraught. For a period of time she was emotionally unavailable to this child, and her sudden emotional absence frightened and over-whelmed him.

THE TWO-TRAUMA MECHANISM:

In the above examples, there was a major separation from a "most important person" in the present—just prior to the acute psychoses—which signified the experienced separation from the "most important person" in the distant past during infancy. Each had a fiance who moved away two to three months before the bizarre reality and behavior was detected. This same sequence was found in the *initial* psychotic episode of nearly all 300 cases of schizophrenia evaluated over the 25 year period, provided the history was known. A trauma in the present, which was in some way similar to the trauma in the distant past, preceded a **partial** shift to the perceptions/reality/feelings/behavior that existed at the precise time/age of the earlier trauma. In each case, it was a major separation from an important person or group that preceded the partial return to the mental/emotional/physiological gestalt that existed at the time of the perceived threat of separation from the mother during infancy.

The loss of an important relationship has been recognized in the PTSD literature as being one of the most profound life stressors (Williams & Siegel, 1989; Holmes, 1967; Meisner, 1977; Lindeman, 1944; and Schmale, 1958). Similarly, the profound effects of early separation of the infant from the mother has been noted by Bowlby (1969, 1973, 1984), Spitz (1945), Reite et al. (1981), Harlow (1958, 1965, 1971, 1979), Cichetti (1984), and MacLean (1973, 1985). Mizukamia (1987) discovered an immediate decrease in skin temperature of the infant upon separation from the mother, indicating stress, and van der Kolk (1988) summarizes the findings of biochemical changes that result from early separation experiences (Coe, 1978; Brown et al., 1982; Kraemer, 1984; Konner, 1982; Tennes, 1982; Landenslager, 1985; Bunny, 1984; Mason et al., 1985; Kolb, 1987; van der Kolk, 1985). Dr. Charles Nemeroff (1993) provides remarkable data demonstrating long term reduction of pituitary production of cortico stimulating factors (CSF) in persons who experienced early separation from their mothers, and he attributes the development of depression to the decreased cortico stimulating factors set in motion by the early separation from the mother.

In summary, early infant separation from the mother—throughout the psychological and biological literature—is described as having a profound and enduring effect.   While the literature acknowledges the early separation experience as being very traumatic and having a lasting effect, we take the concept one step further: Our finding is that all or nearly all infant trauma has one common denominator, which is a relative degree of physical or emotional separation from the mother, as experienced by the infant.

Subsequent life stressors are also major separations. In the former *DSM III-R*, nearly every Axis IV acute event stressor, listed for adults, adolescents or children, is separation. Nowhere, however is a connection made between the current loss/separation and the perceived threat of separation from the mother during infancy.

The mechanism of the shift from a perceived trauma in the present to a similar perceived trauma in the past is thought to be a survival mechanism that has gone awry or, more accurately, is maladaptive. The creature flashes back, or automatically returns, to the same mind/brain/reality/feelings/behavior/chemistry and physiology that existed at the moment of the earlier trauma, and which enabled it to survive the first time. This is a basic survival mechanism. If a gazelle escapes the attack of a lion, the next time the lion attacks, the gazelle—in order to increase its chance for survival—must do exactly what enabled it to survive the first time.

Many ask why this maladaptive survival mechanism is not eliminated through natural selection. The answer is easily understood: *The mechanism itself*—i.e., shifting to the response that enabled the creature to survive the first time (which becomes an automatic, knee-jerk "learned" response)—must work to favor survival of the species more often than not, so the *mechanism* survives even when the results are deleterious in the one percent who have schizophrenia. Schizophrenia and PTSD from trauma in later life are examples in which this survival mechanism is maladaptive.

This mechanism applies to all species, including the human species. For example, a man who fought too long in the front lines during World War II was rabbit hunting 20 years later when someone from across the field accidentally pelleted him with birdshot. Instantly, he spun around and fired five rounds at gut level. His mind raced back to a **similar** time when he was walking across a field toting a gun and was shot at, and he responded in the identical fashion that enabled him to survive the first time.

The reference to a trauma in the present returning the person to a trauma in the distant past, which appears throughout this text, is a shorthand means of referring to a highly complex mental/emotional/biochemical/physiological/neuroanatomic and phylogenetic mechanism: The initial trauma is highly charged emotionally, stirring the infant's fears of abandonment and death, along with feelings of pain and sadness, overwhelming anxiety and despair. This leads to an emotional/mental/physiological gestalt, combined with biochemical change in the particular phylogenetically older structures of the brain that are active at the specific age traumatized. This includes biochemical changes involved in memory. The emotional gestalt may continue to grow and expand, to any degree, as an isolated core nucleus of consciousness in an early developmental region of the brain. Similarly, the non trauma-related portions of the brain continue to grow and develop, to varying degrees, but remain separate from the early trauma site/core nucleus of consciousness. If the early core nucleus remains relatively more active and the later developmental regions of the brain relatively less active, this may account for a decrease in brain volume and an increase in the negative symptoms of schizophrenia.

Decades after the original trauma, a similar trauma precipitates a similar gestalt that indexes to the original "memory"/gestalt and stimulates the same neuroanatomical site that is then reactivated but not consciously remembered. Once the original site is activated, it may perseverate as an epileptogenic focal point (Paul MacLean's terminology, personal correspondence, 1984) —which allows for recurrent acute episodes with little additional stimulation or provocation.

EASE OF REACTIVATION:

The principle of easy reactivation once the core nucleus of consciousness/neuro-anatomical site initially has been activated, applies not just to schizophrenia, but to major depression, bipolar disorder, anxiety and panic attacks, alcohol and drug dependence, and delayed post-traumatic stress disorders of any type. When the early site/nucleus of consciousness is active, the person literally lives **partially** in the earlier timeframe, with gross distortions of perception/reality/behavior which have specificity to the age and brain site that was active at the time of the original trauma. Further evidence and elaboration of the neuroanatomical and biological shift is described in Chapter VI.

The discovery and formulation of the two trauma mechanism provides a new window for therapeutic intervention and a rational effective means of prevention.

3

Inescapable Shock

In inescapable shock (Seligman, 1969), when animals are shocked but are free to escape, the ones that initially had been restrained return to the same helpless behavior of the earlier shock, while others that initially had not been restrained are able to escape. This, too, is the same survival mechanism gone awry, and is a sub-category of the two trauma mechanism. The creature returns to the earlier biological response as an automatic means of handling an emergency situation. Most often this enables the creature to survive, but with the precondition of inescapable shock the mechanism becomes maladaptive. This particular survival mechanism is so basic that it may apply to the entire animal kingdom and may have application to the plant kingdom as well. According to Darwin (1859), to become an adaptive mechanism the behavioral response need only result in survival more often than it results in death.

The inescapable shock model applies not just to laboratory animals, but to patients in every day practice as well. Four recent examples illustrate this particularly well: A 60 year old woman complained of a phobia for rats, mice and insects which she had for as long as she could remember. She attributed the phobia to a large rat chewing on her forehead when she was lying in a bassinet at age 6 months. At that time all she could do was scream for her mother, who came and chased the rat away. Sixty years later, during an eye movement trauma desensitization session, she was picturing her worst fear: a large rat jumping in bed with her and chewing on her forehead. At the end of that particular set of eye movements, her verbalized solution was that she would call to her husband and he would chase the rat away! Incredible. After 60 years her mental solution remained the same. All she could think to do was to lie there and call for someone else to chase the rat away—exactly as she did 60 years earlier. This represents a classical example of the inescapable shock model, spanning 60 years and in the human species. After the realization of her faulty mentation, it was easily corrected with the next two sets of eye movements, as she determined she could chase the rat away herself.

The second example is a 5 year 2 month old child who at age 1 year 2 months laid in a hospital crib with an i.v. in her wrist. The i.v. had missed the vein, was infiltrating her wrist and causing a severe chemical burn. The baby was frightened, in pain, and could not get out of the crib to go to her mother. Many years earlier, I had written that paranoia seems to have its peak age of origin at 14 months, and this child was no exception. In addition to an extreme PTSD with flashbacks precipitated by doctors, hospitals, scissors and bandages, she was overly cautious and suspicious. She clung to her mother and studied new persons intently for hours before approaching them. After four years of therapy, approximately 20 hours per year, she finally seemed to be resolving the trauma. Then at age 5 years 2 months, she had just finished her therapy session and was excited about stepping outside and taking a turn at looking through a telescope at the stars while her older sister came in for her therapy session. After 15 minutes, we heard her crying and discovered that when she realized she was alone looking through the telescope, she was afraid and was unable to move—even though her mother was just the other side of the door that was only ten feet away. The experience returned her to the 14 month trauma during which she had been frightened and unable to move because of being caged in a crib. This time, immediately upon being returned to her mother, she curled up in a fetal position in her mother's lap, tucking her head under her mother's chin, exactly as she did following the original trauma.

The third example of inescapable shock is from the October 4, 1992 Bijlmermeer disaster (McKenzie, 1993a). When the Boeing 747 hit the 10 story apartment building and the jet fuel exploded, many residents could not escape because the building shifted, jamming the doors. One such apartment contained three adults who were evaluated by the first author, seven months after the disaster. At the sound of thunder or a low flying airplane, all three run to the door of their new apartment and cannot open it. A fourth resident—who was not present in the disaster—has to open the door for them.

From another airline crash, the Sahsa Boeing 737 in Managua, Nicaragua, July 18, 1993 (McKenzie, 1993b), the first author identified one very unique case of inescapable shock among the 51 victims he evaluated. A 43 year old woman who injured her jaw and could not speak at the time of the crash, is unable to move her jaw during flashbacks—even though it is well healed. This example demonstrates that the immobility found in inescapable shock can apply to a body part as well as to the whole body.

The immobility at the second trauma in all the above examples is classical for the inescapable shock model, and only the understanding of the mechanism has changed. Instead of "learned helplessness," it is regarded as maladaptive survival behavior. As part of the survival mechanism, the creature behaves and does exactly what it did the first time in order to survive once more.

The "freeze" response, which is sometimes seen in adult homo sapiens in lieu of the fight or flight response, is at times a similar return to an earlier inescapable shock from infancy. One woman at Bijlmermeer was eight months pregnant when the disaster occurred. The fetus stopped moving in utero and no more movements were detected until after delivery. Will this infant respond by "freezing" later in life? How does this affect its **temperamental patterns**? A 13 year old girl was in the kitchen at the time of the explosion. She opened the door to run to the living room where her older brother was standing, but the living room was no longer there. At interview, this girl exhibited a "jungle awareness." She did not move; she sat crouched like a creature hiding from some overwhelming danger. Only her eyes moved, scanning the room with nervous hypervigilance. Is this a source/mechanism of numbing in PTSD? Or a source of flat affect in schizophrenia?

We have digressed from the discussion of inescapable shock. Once pointed out in real life examples, it is easier to understand how the mechanism works, and it is clear that it represents a maladaptive survival mechanism. In the field of psychiatry, the application of inescapable shock has been limited to the study of depression. To see this simply as a learned maladaptive mechanism does not capture the entire picture. All, or nearly all, serious mental illness may be the result of a return to an earlier means of survival, whether that means of survival was freezing in place, combat readiness, or maladaptive pessimism. The frozen-in-place response occurs when the individual was frozen in place the first time he survived a severe traumatic experience—whether he was frozen in place because of being too young to move, or because he was strapped down, or because a "freeze" response was automatically elicited the first time—possibly representing a phylogenetic return to an adaptive mechanism of an earlier species.

4

Flashbacks, and Other Early Trauma

FLASHBACKS:

Flashbacks are the partial or complete return to the initial trauma, which can be precipitated by any stimuli that *signify* the original trauma. This mechanism had not been applied to early infant trauma because early trauma had not been clearly identified (van der Kolk, 1988). Furthermore, the realities of infancy are so strikingly different from the realities of the adult, that when they recur they are mistakenly attributed to *unreality* instead of *earlier* reality. This makes the source of behavior more difficult to identify. When carefully scrutinized, each piece of disturbed reality/perception/behavior of the psychotic is related to that of the infant at the age originally traumatized. As we later explore a series of early realities that manifest clinically in the adult schizophrenic, certain unmistakable landmarks will begin to appear.

OTHER EARLY TRAUMAS:

Various early traumas have been identified, in addition to the birth of a sibling, the emotional upset of the mother, and the unique and unusual examples of inescapable shock cited above. One such early trauma, that surfaced through cumulative histories over the 25 year period, is moving from one dwelling to another. While the mother busies herself trying to make the new place look like home, the infant may become frightened as he quickly senses the change in her priori-

33

ties. Catastrophes may cause the infant to feel threatened: the family may lose its home or the father might lose his job, a close relative or parent might die or there may be a serious illness in the family. With any catastrophe, the infant may lose some of the attention from its mother. In addition to emotional separation from the mother, there can be physical separations as well, such as the mother or infant being hospitalized or the mother going on vacation, or even sometimes going to work. The sudden absence of the mother, if not carefully attenuated, easily can serve as a traumatic experience to the infant, particularly if this is accompanied by pain, such as from a surgical procedure, or if it had already experienced earlier trauma, such as birth trauma (Grof, 1985; Mednick et al., 1987; Dykes, Mednick et al., 1992; Cannon, Mednick et al., 1993).

(The cumulative nature of trauma is already known to the PTSD literature: Burgess and Holstrom (1979), Hendin et al. (1983), Helzer (1987) all note that prior trauma predisposes one to PTSD. Helzer et al. (1987) and Hough et al. (1989) found that antecedent emotional problems predispose persons to PTSD. Pynoos and Nader (1988) noted that effects of repeated trauma are additive. Doyle and Bauer (1989) refer to "layered trauma," Kahn (1963) to "cumulative trauma" and Kris (1956) to "strain trauma." Freud (1926) noted that anxiety predisposes one to trauma. The present authors add to this the concept that not only is a trauma greater because of prior trauma or anxiety, *but this same isolated trauma-related core nucleus of consciousness can continue to grow and expand as subsequent nightmares, frightening experiences, and conscious and unconscious flashbacks continue to feed into it and seal over*). (See diagrams A–E.)

Sometimes the infant is not only separated from the mother, but is placed in a new surrounding with unfamiliar caregivers. This can be even more frightening. While the most frequent single cause of schizophrenia, in as many as one-third of the cases, was found to be the birth of a sibling in the first 24 months, this may not apply to future generations. Presently more than 50 percent of women with one year old babies are placing them in daycare centers. The results remain unrecognized and untabulated, but there is a potential danger. Whether the risk is greater or lesser than the preliminary findings among those with siblings 24 months younger or less, is yet to be determined. If the results are as dramatically adverse as anticipated, then the widespread use of daycare may be a greater hazard than people realize, and the apparent financial advantage may be more of a disadvantage to family and to nation.

Another early trauma is the "one year nanny program." Here a substitute caregiver is supplied for the infant in the home for one year and at the end of that time she leaves. Because visas to the United States are granted for one year, a vast number of infants have been subjected to this trauma. Later in life, if traumatized sufficiently to precipitate a mental disorder, the person will have an illness that corresponds to his particular age and reality during infancy when the visa expired.

5

Earlier Realities as Seen in the Adult

NON-SPECIFIC INFANT BEHAVIOR/REALITIES:

The behavior of our schizophrenic patients was found to relate to infant behavior. Some could be attributed to a specific month of origin while other behavior spanned a longer period of time during infancy. A full grown man, sitting in the middle of the floor screaming "Mommy, Mommy, Mommy," is reexperiencing a moment of trauma from his infancy, but his behavior is not specific enough to identify a particular month.

A grown woman, squealing with delight, running nude through a lawn sprinkler in the front yard, is exhibiting perfectly normal behavior,—but transposed from a much earlier time. Something caused her to return to an earlier behavioral age, but once more, this particular behavior alone does not reveal a specific month.

LANDMARK REALITIES:

The following are clinical vignettes of experiences of seriously disturbed individuals which allow us to identify an age specific reality. These are samples to illustrate a return to a specific early time, and this is not an attempt to provide a complete list.

One man was found upside down in a fetal position trying to force his head through a toilet bowl. Since birth can be a painful, near-death experience to some infants, and since terrifying moments leave indelible impressions to which persons return, we believe it possible that this man actually could have been reexperiencing a particularly frightening birth experience.

Less obvious is the woman who, while holding a rational conversation, experienced pain around her face, head, neck and shoulders. Careful clinical observation and assessment revealed that the pain occurred every six minutes. There is no medical reason for this to occur every six minutes. History revealed that her mother was given general anesthesia during delivery. We presume this would have been given when the mother was experiencing her greatest difficulty, and based on moment-of-trauma specificity observed in others, we suspect this could have been when the mother's contractions were six minutes apart. If indeed she returned to the part of her mind/brain she was using at birth, then it was only a partial return because she was able to carry on a normal conversation. We suspect that nearly all children during the first year of life demonstrate *symptoms* of anxiety which appear related to birth. When a T-shirt is pulled over the head of a one year old, for example, it may scream, tense all the muscles in its little body, and turn red as its head is being forced through the neck of the T-shirt. Some one year olds also have anxiety dreams which seem to be about birth (McKenzie, 1982).

One 20 year old man was terrified that he might scratch his face with his fingernails or hit himself in the face with his fist. This would be realistic at age two to three months when the baby is waving its arms around and "clawing" with its fingernails but does not yet have enough control to keep from hurting itself. This young man had been terrified of hurting himself at that age because of having experienced severe trauma, anoxia, and brain damage at birth. He also had been abandoned by his mother at birth and then adopted two weeks later.

Various therapeutic modalities were considered for his treatment. He was obviously caught in a much earlier reality from which he had to return. A trial of medication had not worked and something more dramatic was needed. If a person is having a bad dream, one might shake him to wake him up, and if a person is delirious, one might slap his face. Likewise, when a person is caught in a delusional reality and medication does not suffice, he may need an even more substantial jolt to return him more fully to present reality. This patient required more, and shock treatment was chosen for him.

Part of the rationale for shock treatment related to another observation over the course of the clinical experience: namely, *the mind centers on the point in time where the most imminent threat to survival is experienced.* This may be another survival mechanism that is built into the species and perhaps the entire animal kingdom. This phenomenon was described in the mental hospitals in France during World War II. When patients were told that the soldiers were coming to shoot them, and the hospital doors were opened, the inmates acted in accordance with present adult-brain reality. They began to function as persons without schizophrenia: i.e., instead of being trapped in the early infant part of the mind/brain that was terrified of abandonment and death, there was a shift of activity to the later developmental portion of the mind/brain that was reactivated by terror of imminent slaughter in the present.

In another account, one schizophrenic describes his own technique for bringing himself out of psychosis, which was to mount a fast horse and race through the woods. He had to hang on for dear life, of course, and the danger of falling off—in the present—was more imminent and superseded the perceived danger of abandonment by the mother in the past. This, too, "activated" the present mind/brain/reality to the exclusion of the earlier mind/brain/reality. Koegler & Hicks (1972) describe mental patients suddenly functioning normally during an earthquake. For a short period of time, they were relatively free from their mental disorders.

While there are other explanations as to why shock treatment works, there was no question that it *did* work for this patient who was injured at birth and feared scratching his face. He was very much afraid of shock treatment, but after the first one, he suddenly stopped being afraid that he would scratch his face with his fingernails or hit himself in the face with his fist. That early reality/fear from the first few months of life immediately disappeared. He continued to improve until the third shock treatment, during which he struggled and did not receive the pre-ECT oxygen. As a result, he became a little cyanotic. The next morning he complained of excruciating pain in the head, neck, shoulders and upper back. His tongue protruded slightly from his mouth to the extent that it became dry and fissured. His pain was so intense that the immediate clinical impression was that he had fractured a cervical vertebrae with the last treatment. But more careful observation of him while he was eating revealed that his tongue pushed forward in his mouth causing food to drop out. This is the tongue motion of the infant feeding, prior to taking solid foods. Clinically, therefore, it was determined that the anoxia at the time of the shock treatment returned him to the anoxia at birth, and he returned so completely to that part of the mind/brain/reality that he was re-experiencing the identical pain symptoms and body movements he had at the earlier time, at birth. Thus, instead of an X-ray, he was given the next treatment. The excruciating pain in the head, neck and upper back disappeared as expected, and his tongue retracted to its normal position. After the sixth treatment, the symptoms returned once more and it was learned that the treatment team once more had been unable to give him oxygen prior to the treatment. With the next treatment, these symptoms again disappeared.

COMPARISONS WITH ADULT TRAUMA:

A similar mechanism occurs in patients who are reexperiencing trauma of adult life (as opposed to specific trauma of infancy). For example, one man who had his shoulder crushed three years earlier, suddenly experienced a recurrence of the identical pain when, while watching TV, he saw a tractor trailer back into and crush a man's shoulder. Flashbacks and unconscious flashbacks may account for a portion of phantom limb pain and explain one reason why it is intermittent instead of constant. A person can return partially or nearly completely to any earlier traumatic point in time and reexperience the early memories, feelings and realities. One patient may have even partially reexperienced a coma in the form of a psychomotor seizure. In the initial trauma, she was the passenger in the car her fiance was driving when a tractor trailer pulled out in front of them and her fiance was crushed to death. On impact, she was knocked unconscious and remained in coma for several days. One year later, a tractor trailer ran through an intersection and she swerved her car just in time to miss hitting it. The next thing she was able to recall was turning into her driveway, 20 miles away. The recent near-collision returned her to the first accident and part of her mind returned to the blank, comatose state while another part of her mind drove the car home. This is not altogether different from a part of one's mind/brain being intensely involved in a dream, and another part of the mind/brain having little or no awareness of it upon awakening. It is also similar to the two states of mind in a post hypnotic suggestion, and to the two states of mind in all dissociative disorders.

The flashback that returns an individual to a specific traumatic event in his adult life is basic to PTSD (Lyons et al., 1988; Emery and Smith, 1987; Brett & Ostroff, 1985; Green et al., 1985; Keane & Kaloupeck, 1982). By a somewhat similar process, the neurotic, in stressful situations, returns to earlier feelings, realities and fantasies of childhood and acts them out with others. But the return to a specific moment during infancy has remained less obvious. The infant is the most delicate and vulnerable of all, however, and he/she is totally dependent on the mother. In some institutions infants were found to have a 50 percent chance of dying of anaclitic depression if a previously constant mother figure suddenly was not available (Spitz, 1945, 1975). Many studies indicate that the younger the individual is when the trauma occurs, the more susceptible he is and the more intractable the PTSD becomes. Younger veterans are affected longer (Boros, 1973); younger persons who lose a spouse experience greater PTSD (Williams & Siegel, 1989); the younger the rape victim, the greater the PTSD (Kilpatrick, 1985); children are vulnerable to wider range of stressors (Hyman et al., 1988); children are more vulnerable to less extreme stressors (Pynoos & Eth, 1985; Raifman, 1983; Zelikoff, 1986); younger hostages correlate with more PTSD (van der Ploeg and Kleijn, 1989); younger persons are less able to integrate traumatic memories (Janet, 1919); children are more vulnerable because of the undeveloped nature of their coping mechanisms (Eth & Pynoos, 1985); individuals who were children during the Holocaust are more affected (Gampel, 1988, 1989; Kestenberg, 1982; Kestenberg & Brenner, 1986; Klein, 1974, 1983), and children are more vulnerable to disorganization in the face of stress (van der Kolk, 1988).

The pattern is clear, and the infant is the youngest of all. Spitz (1945, 1975, 1983) noted the earlier and the more prolonged the separation from the mother (after capacity for object relationship is developed, age 4–6 months), the more severe the trauma, the more profound the depression and the higher the incidence of death. The trauma of early separation, or anything that causes the infant to fear it, conceivably represents the maximal stressor known to mankind. Couple this with the fact that an individual can return to a specific moment in time, and the *un*realities of schizophrenia become recognized instead as *earlier* realities of infancy. Thus, it becomes understandable when a schizophrenic falls down and experiences the reality that the floor came up and hit him in the head. He has returned to the particular age that correlates with that psychological reality. It becomes understandable why a schizophrenic patient moves both arms in unison like a baby, or when he walks with elbows extended laterally to maintain his balance as he did when he first began to walk, etc.

OTHER EXAMPLES OF AGE SPECIFIC REALITIES:

Correlating particular emotional symptoms with age at birth of the next sibling allows for an accurate clinical post diction regarding the age at which the original trauma occurred, based on the clinical symptoms of the patient (McKenzie 1981, 1984, 1986a, 1986b, 1992).

One patient, for example, hung his mother's cat because it supposedly was answering the telephone. A primary symptom of experiencing the reality that animals can talk is derived from a time when the child can say a few words but not enough to realize that animals cannot talk. Clinically this is probably the mental reality of a child age 14 months. History confirmed this clinical post diction when it was learned that the patient had a sister 14 months younger. His first psychotic episode began after he left a wife in Vietnam. This separation from "the most important person" returned him to the original separation from "the most important person," when his sister was born and his mother "left" him.

Age 14 months also coincides with a peak age for later development of the most rigid, extreme form of paranoia, which was found in this man. At age 12 months, the baby takes his first steps. By age 14 months, he is traveling everywhere, and the whole world (his mother) watches him vigilantly and follows him wherever he goes (so that he does not fall down the stairs or put hairpins in electrical outlets, etc.).

Trauma at age 17 months often corresponds with the formerly common diagnosis of simple schizophrenia. Perceptual and cognitive object permanence is achieved by 18 months (Piaget, 1936). According to Mahler (1979), "By the 18th month, the junior toddler seems to be at the height of the process of dealing with his continuously experienced physical separation from the mother." Just prior to achieving this, the infant is wandering into the next room and peeking back to see if the mother is still there. Like a chick that pecks the hardest at the shell just before breaking out, the person at age 17 months is tugging the hardest at the boundaries between himself and the mother. Consequently, persons who under stress return to that mental stage often become wanderers, forever leaving and returning to their motherland. One person who had a sibling 17 months younger and who was not overtly schizophrenic, had returned partially to the earlier reality. From Philadelphia, he moved to France, then to Maine then to Germany.

Not everyone traumatized at age 17 months becomes a wanderer, but since first noting a correlation approximately ten years ago, three more "wanderers" were found who had younger siblings within the first two years of life. In each case the sibling was 17 months younger. While the total number is small, the narrow age range and the exclusivity points toward significance. Carefully controlled studies are needed to determine the peak age of origin and the age range of this and all other symptoms related to infant trauma.

In 1988 a woman brought her 28 year old daughter for therapy. She supposedly had schizophrenia for 12 years. Subtle clinical clues, in particular her affect and degree of warmth, more nearly matched her symptoms with those of persons traumatized at age 20 months—which correlated with disorders in the schizo-affective range. (Note: We refer to a schizoaffective range, between 18 and 24 months of origin. Persons who meet *DSM IV* criteria for schizoaffective disorder most likely were traumatized during this time interval. But when we refer to a schizoaffective range, we are more inclusive than the *DSM IV* criteria. There is something qualitatively different about persons traumatized after 18 months of age; they exhibit more affect, greater warmth and they appear healthier. These qualities are detected immediately. In the earlier part of the schizoaffective range, especially at 19 and 20 months, there are a number of patients who would meet the *DSM IV* criteria for paranoid schizophrenia, but these individuals are qualitatively different from paranoid schizophrenics of age 13 to 15 months origin. Many or most persons with paranoid schizophrenia from age 13 to 15 months would fail to meet *DSM-IV* criteria for paranoid schizophrenia because of having flat affect. We eagerly await more data on schizoaffective patients and do not yet rule out the possibility of two separate early traumas. This possibility still holds true for bipolar disorders as well.)

With this particular patient, as part of therapeutic style, the first author said, within minutes of meeting her: "You don't have schizophrenia; you missed it by two months. The origin of schizophrenia is in the first 18 months of life [schizophrenia in the non-schizoaffective range] and something happened to you at age 20 months." (This blunt, authoritative approach has therapeutic value, particularly when it is validated during the session. It adds convincing support to the psychodynamic explanations.) Later during this particular session, the clinical and etiologic impression was confirmed when it was learned that the young lady had a brother who was 20 months younger. (This session is on tape.)

Post diction appears increasingly possible concerning the timing of trauma. Another woman called on the telephone, crying hysterically, in a deep depression with extreme self-hatred and guilt. Her intensity of this emotion and degree of self-blame matched that which clinically peaks in persons traumatized at age 2 years 2 months. When asked if there were a sibling two years two months younger, she said there was a brother 2 years younger. After comparing the birth dates, it was 2 years 2 months and 1 day.

After years of clinical experience, our cumulative impression is that through study and practice it is possible to identify the age of traumatic experience usually to within one month. While the post dictive precision is a repeated finding, not all the parameters used can be described. Some are clear and obvious while others are subtle and ill defined. Nonetheless, the age specific early reality/behavior seen later in life may be as precise or even more precise than the developmental stages of the infant. Developmental stages may change after trauma, but the trauma fixes the original developmental stage and the site in the brain. The accuracy of the post diction will be put to the test, with no attachment to any particular result, and future clinical study will continue to identify and refine the age specific parameters. It is clear that the mind returns to the *moment* of the trauma, since the reality and behavior of the patient matches the reality and behavior at the time the original trauma occurred. It remains to be proven how accurate the clinical post dictions are, but preliminary pilot study data supports the broad categories of the cumulative observations (McKenzie 1986).

While there are developmental landmarks found in the adult schizophrenic that "mark the spot" or the precise time of the trauma during infancy, sometimes the landmarks are partially obscured because realities vary in each infant's environment. For example, some infants are reared in a crib and therefore are not "followed" as vigilantly everywhere they go. Some may have nervous, watchful or critical mothers, as opposed to relaxed, accepting mothers. This alters the experience within the developmental stage, and therefore within the developmental reality of the schizophrenic. The developmental landmarks also can be obscured by the clinical course of the disease process, by multiplicity of trauma, by individual developmental differences over the lifetime of the person, and by character traits carried forward from various earlier periods of time. But the developmental landmarks are still present—and they still relate to the peak moment of terror—even though they are partially obscured.

GARY HEIDNIK'S AGE SPECIFIC REALITIES:

In the notorious case of Gary Heidnik, who chained a number of women in his basement because he wanted babies, a post dictive statement was notarized, based on newspaper accounts, prior to even meeting Mr. Heidnik. The statement said that Gary Heidnik was using the mind/brain/reality of age 18 months and, therefore, it was predicted that his brother would be 18 months younger. This prediction was one month off. But had he been evaluated clinically first, the estimate would have been 17 months, because there was a certain peculiarity and oddity about his behavior not reported in the newspaper. Also, it was later learned that he too had been somewhat of a wanderer, moving from Ohio to California to Germany in the Service and then to Philadelphia. After hundreds of hours of study of Gary Heidnik, it was possible to identify approximately 40 bits of reality and behavior that were related exclusively to the reality and behavior of the earlier time. This is detailed in a proposed book, "When the Baby Kills" (McKenzie and Sullivan, unpublished).

From Gary Heidnik's history it was clear that his first psychosis was facilitated by a near-lethal dose of hallucinogenic substance given to him while he was in Germany in the military—at the time when the CIA reportedly was conducting human experimentation on our servicemen. Subsequent psychotic episodes followed rejections and separations from important people, and also followed renewed contact with the persons who were present at the time of the original trauma, i.e., original family members.

After approximately 25 hospitalizations over the course of as many years, Mr. Heidnik had one experience that took him deeper and more completely into his psychosis than ever before. He had married a woman from the Philippines who left him soon after she became pregnant. He immediately made a suicide attempt and was hospitalized for more than one month in the VA Hospital in Coatesville, Pennsylvania. She returned to him once more, but he was extremely difficult to live with, and she was forced to leave again. In October, 1986, he received a postcard from her stating that their son had been born September 15. This returned him to the first time the most important woman in the world "left" him and had a baby. To the 17 month old, there are big people and little people. Big people control the little people. Big people come and go as they please and little people cannot. Big people punish little people. When Heidnik's 17 month brain took command, he reversed all this. By Thanksgiving, 1986 he captured his first victim and chained her in his basement.

While the adult portion of his mind coexisted with the reawakened infant part, it was the infant part of the mind/brain/reality that was in charge. No woman was ever going to leave him again. No one was ever going to take his babies away again (this was the fourth time he fathered a baby who was taken away). When the infant portion of the brain is sufficiently activated and decides that mommy is never going to leave him again, the adult portion of the brain becomes subservient to the new command center, and it drives the car to buy the chains. And while the adult brain knows how to do things the infant brain cannot, it is no longer in charge. It is only semi-present, as in a dream state.

Heidnik noticed that the one girl, Sandy, was not eating. He became very concerned about her and stuffed two pieces of bread in her mouth like a child would do with a pet bird. When he returned, she was not moving. He was stunned with disbelief. He had no idea what happened to Sandy, but realized that he must dispose of her,—otherwise someone would stop his plan. And how does the infant make something disappear? By putting it in the mouth....

Body parts were fed to the dogs that dropped bones upstairs, downstairs, out in the yard, and even in front of the other victims in the basement. Other parts of the body were ground up and fed to the victims. Arms and legs were neatly wrapped in freezer paper and labeled. These were *to be fed to the babies when they were weaned from the breast*! To a child psychoanalyst, this thought clearly originates from the mind of the infant. As in Lewin's Oral Triad (Lewin, 1946, 1958), the infant has three wishes: to eat, to be eaten and to sleep. The infant first goes through the sucking phase, but then shortly after developing teeth, begins to have the wish to devour the mother (Erikson, 1950). This thought is believed to be present in all infants and becomes apparent if an adult jokingly says to a two year old, "I'm going to gobble you up." The child may react with terror because this thought touches his own.

Of equal interest is what happened to bring Gary Heidnik out of the acute psychosis. Shortly after he was apprehended, he was beaten by other inmates and was fearful of being killed. Since the mind focuses on the point in time where there is the most **imminent** threat to survival, the threat of being killed by the inmates helped him shift away from the part of the mind and brain that was caught up with the fear of abandonment and death at age 17 months, and he became more adult reality oriented.

Heidnik's recall of the four months with the women in the cellar is very hazy and dream-like. In fact, he can recognize only the picture of the first girl, Sandy, because he knew her very well prior to his acute psychotic episode. Images of the other women had been recorded primarily by the reawakened infant brain, and his adult mind/brain was not present in sufficient *density* to record their appearances. When he returned to his adult mind/brain/reality, he was sickened by the occurrences that had taken place, as these actions were incongruous with his adult mind. He became ill and nearly vomited when asked about digging the girls' ear drums out with a screwdriver. This is parallel to a nightmare that a normal individual might have wherein he injures or kills people he cares for. At some level in the dream he might know that it is wrong to do this, but another part of his mind is in charge and does it nonetheless. On awakening, the person can be upset by what he did during the dream that is incongruous with the morals of his rational (adult) mind.

FURTHER EXAMPLES OF AGE SPECIFIC REALITIES:

Clinical symptoms repeatedly identify accurately the age at the time of the original trauma. An important age for non psychotic depression, for example, is 2 years 6 months. A classical example is Marilyn Monroe, whose mother went to a mental hospital when Marilyn was 2-1/2 years old. At age 2 years 6 months, the toddler experiences the reality that "mommy went away and left me." And since the toddler sees the mother grandly, as if a goddess at that age, it blames the self and hates the self, in terms of the 2-1/2 year old's concepts: bad, ugly, unlovable. Marilyn's entire life was a desperate attempt to make herself beautiful and lovable, but in the end she continued to experience the 2-1/2 year old reality of being unlovable once more.

Recently, a woman came for treatment and the age of origin was not totally clear. Her psychosis began ten years earlier when her fiance left her. She was extremely regressed and sat eating her lunch while urinating in her clothing. A urologist thought that she had a bladder disorder. But careful observation revealed that soiling her clothing was ego-syntonic and seemed natural to her. Clinically this meant that it was not a problem of bladder control. She was regressed to an earlier time when it was normal for the baby in the highchair to casually wet its diaper while eating.

At lunch she filled a hoagie roll with egg salad and pushed it against her face, with the upper lip extended upward and the lower lip downward. She proceeded to make short, rapid chewing motions with her jaw as she slowly shoved the food into her mouth. Clinically this was a partial reexperiencing of an early feeding situation, but neither the wetting of the diaper nor the feeding behavior were specific enough to identify a particular early age. She was quite capable of expressing affect, however, which narrowed the range of function to somewhere between 18 and 24 months. She also had some depression and paranoia which were consistent with the amount that can be present in the schizo-affective range. Additionally, she exhibited hypomanic behavior at times and had been treated with Lithium in the past. Although clinical experience with manic depressive psychosis was insufficient to be conclusive, in regard to age of origin, there were indications that part of the disorder may relate to trauma at age 1 year 10 months. Thus, her background was searched to learn what might have happened to her at age 1 year 10 months. She knew that her mother was hospitalized for a nervous breakdown just prior to her turning 2 years old, and we thought that this might have happened near the Christmas holidays. Since her birth date was in February, this would set the age of origin of her illness at approximately 1 year 10 months. This type of data is of little value for research, however, because it does not provide a precise time. Furthermore, the mother could have been upset for a month or two prior to hospitalization, and she might have been similarly upset on numerous other occasions. Thus, once more, the birth of a sibling is a preferable parameter because the exact age is known, and there is not another sibling born a few months before or after.

RELATIONSHIP BETWEEN DURATION AND SEVERITY OF ILLNESS:

In the above example, even though the woman was in the schizo-affective range, she acted extremely regressed. While usually schizophrenia of earlier traumatic origin was found to be more severe, this woman was much sicker than most persons who were traumatized several months earlier. This is because she had been allowed to remain deep in her psychosis for 10 years. With PTSD it is preferable to treat as soon as possible after the trauma. This is noted throughout the PTSD literature: Raphiel (1977), Horowitz (1976), van der Kolk & Ducey (1984), Pynoos & Nadar (1988), van der Ploeg & Kleijn (1989), Kardiner (1941), Krystal (1978), Green et al. (1985), Stretch (1985, 1986, 1989), Talbot (1990), and Terr (1994). With delayed onset PTSD, it is important to bring about an immediate recovery from the sudden, acute state. This is especially true in regard to delayed PTSD from infancy. Our clinical experience with delayed PTSD from infancy has shown that the longer the person is allowed to remain in the infant part of the mind/brain/reality, the more it encompasses his total existence, and the more difficult it is to treat. With the McKenzie Method (McKenzie, 1981) for treatment of serious emotional disorders, great effort is made to get the person out of the infant mind/brain/reality as quickly as possible, as completely as possible, and for as long as possible. An attempt is made to correct every trace and vestige of the earlier mind/brain/reality. This helps to remove connections with the earlier mind/brain/reality, and to prevent vestiges of the illness from becoming a permanent part of the personality/character.

6

Biological Shift to Earlier Brain, Physiology, Chemistry

NEUROPHYSIOLOGICAL AND NEUROANATOMICAL COUNTERPARTS:

Everything described thus far, as taking place in earlier parts of the mind, appears to have physical counterparts in the structure and the activity of the brain itself. We note that in schizophrenia there is markedly less activity in the prefrontal cortex (Boffey, 1986; Schneck, 1986), which contains some of the most advanced or "human" portions of the brain, the part of the brain that morphologically has been used by physical anthropologists to distinguish humans from lower animals with sloping foreheads. (See Diagram "F" in Appendix.)

The prefrontal cortex is the area of brain that becomes most active during cognitive processes in normal individuals. The area of greatest activity in schizophrenics shifts to various diffuse sites in the brain. This shift may be sub-cortical, or it may be to phylogenetically earlier locations, but there is a definite shift, as current information is processed in accordance with the reality/feelings/behavior of an earlier time. While the higher cortex may be functioning well enough to drive a car, for example, the person might be guided by a 14 month reality that says "everyone is watching and following me everywhere I go." As a result of the relative inactivity in the prefrontal cortex and other higher developmental centers of the brain of the schizophrenic, an atrophy develops.

Atrophy of the more highly developed regions of the brain in schizophrenia has been recognized and described for more than 150

51

years (Crow, 1990). It is reported by Andreason et al. (1986), Barta et al., R. Brown et al., Hoffman et al., Mathew et al., Pearlson et al. (1989), Suddath et al. (1989), and at the May, 1994 American Psychiatric Association meetings in Philadelphia, there were more than two dozen presentations that noted specific areas of atrophy or disuse in the more highly developed structures. These included papers by McCarley et al., Shenton et al., Pearlson et al., Goldman-Rakic, Nasrallah, Arnold, Nestor, Shedlack, Russell, O'Donnell, Niznikiewicz, Wu, Rossi, RC Gur, RE Gur, Dewan, and Hokama.

The authors hold the view that the shift in brain activity from the developed to the more primitive structures, leads to *disuse* and ultimately **disuse atrophy** of the more advanced areas of the brain, which is the same as would occur in any other part of the body not being used. Thus the result of the disuse is disuse atrophy and cognitive impairment, and eventually the atrophy itself contributes to the cognitive impairment. A large portion of cognitive impairment reverses in many schizophrenic patients when they separate from original nuclear family and return to adult mentation. Clinically this was observed repeatedly over the last 25 years, and prompted the first author, more than 20 years ago, to postulate that perhaps the disuse atrophy reverses as well. Both the atrophy and its probable reversal were described in "The Anatomy and Psychodynamics of Psychoses" (McKenzie, 1984). The reversal of brain atrophy also was predicted for alcoholics who attained sobriety because clinically alcoholism was seen as a parallel process. While these predictions seemed unlikely, since central nervous system damage is irreversible, the reversal of the cognitive impairment was a repeated clinical observation. Was the disuse atrophy, therefore, just a softening of brain tissue or a partial reduction of myelin? (We are aware that **destruction** of CNS myelin is considered irreversible.) Finally, in 1985, there was confirmation that the atrophy in alcoholics reverses after six months of sobriety (Carlen, et al.). The authors continue to expect the same will be found in some forms of schizophrenia, when the disease process is reversed early in the course of the illness, and the before and after measurements are taken.

One of the clearest arguments for disuse atrophy relates to the development of the primary language center of the brain. According to Timothy Crow (1990), there is massive development of the left posterior superior temporal gyrus when language development is at its peak. The development is so extensive that the sulci elongate, and the differences between the two hemispheres can be seen on gross examination of the brain or even on MRI. Since we know, from cumulative retrospective analysis, that the schizophrenic returns to the mind/behavior/reality that existed prior to the massive development of language, and since we know that the language center—which develops subsequent to that early mind/behavior/reality—is atrophied proportionately more than any other region of the brain in schizophrenia (Crow), we can deduce that the patient is returning *to the area of the brain* he was using at the earlier time, to the partial exclusion of the language center—which then undergoes disuse atrophy.

In addition to the inactivity and the atrophy in the prefrontal cortex and the left posterior superior temporal gyrus, and in addition to the increased activity in various other areas of the brain of schizophrenics, aberrant neuronal pathways develop in the hippocampus, which stands phylogenetically between the old mammalian and the reptilian portions of the brain. Notwithstanding the principles of neotany, "Ontogeny recapitulates phylogeny" remains a powerful principle that likely does not stop suddenly at birth. While at least some of the old mammalian brain must be operating at birth in order for there to be a sucking reflex, some of the earliest structures of the brain initially are more active as well. This accounts in part for age specific learning abilities (Doman, 1974, 1984; Pearce, 1977, 1985). Later developmental structures or regions of the brain sequentially become more active as the center of thought processes while the young mind/brain is progressing through developmental stages. The trauma that sets the stage for the later development of schizophrenia can occur anywhere along this continuum. This explains why not all schizophrenics are using the same areas of the brain. DeLisi (1994) notes that the morphological brain defects in schizophrenia vary from patient to patient, some being developmental and others occurring after the onset of the illness, and she calls for more research to determine which factors are genetic and which are secondary to the illness process or the environment of the patient. It is our view the age of the infant (and possibly the fetus) at the time of the trauma determines the specific developmental region of the brain affected. Thus, the positron emission tomography (PET) and other physiological studies should be scrutinized and categorized according to age of original trauma. The authors predict that composite PET scans, lined up according to age at the time of original trauma, will reveal a progression of areas of activity from the phylogenetically old to the more developmentally advanced regions of the brain, and that this progression will continue through the psychotic and non-psychotic depressions.

Crow (1994) recognizes a continuum from schizophrenia to schizoaffective to bipolar manic depressive to unipolar depressive psychosis, but he is searching for genetic implications. We have identified the same continuum, possibly beginning with autism and borderlines, then progressing through the schizophrenias, from the bizarre to the tenable, and from the inappropriate and flat to the not-so-flat affect, with schizoaffective and bipolar II overlapping next (here we have insufficient data), followed by major depression with psychotic features and then major depression without psychotic features—all sequentially arranged according to age of trauma.

Brain chemistries and neuro transmitters also are expected to vary because the reactivated phylogenetically older regions of the brain produce proportionately more of the important neuro-transmitters, and because the mental processes of the reawakened earlier brain involve themes of intense emotion, such as fear, pain and despair. Thus, the authors believe that the schizophrenic returns partially to the mind/brain/reality/feeling/behavior/chemistry and physiology of a specific earlier time.

The recent monozygote twin studies (Suddath, 1990) came as no surprise. The brains of those with schizophrenia were atrophied in comparison to their identical twin counterparts. This is what the authors had predicted for more than 20 years. If one identical twin becomes a body builder and the other anorexic, would not the bodies be different? Biological change is seen primarily as a result of function. This includes biochemistry, neurophysiology, neuro transmission, aberrant neuronal pathways, neuroanatomical augmentation and atrophy, neuroanatomical sites of activity, etc.

While the authors consider function to be predominantly responsible for biological change, most researchers continue to regard biological change as being responsible for differences in function and behavior. If biological change is viewed as a result of the return to a terrifying early moment in time, and if it is seen as a natural result of the disease process, then this would explain why biological change is found in such great abundance.

While our findings identify function as primary and biological change as secondary, this is not viewed as exclusive or one directional: genetic predisposition, gestational viral infections, obstetrical complications, and early developmental structural change can and do impact on function.

POSITIVE & NEGATIVE SYMPTOMS:
THE TIMOTHY CROW THEORY AND OUR VIEW:

Positive versus negative symptoms, according to Andreason et al. (1990), were first identified by Kraepelin (1919) and referred to as florid symptoms versus symptoms marked by losses and deficits. Bleuler (1950) distinguished between fundamental and accessory symptoms. By far the most detailed description is made by Andreason in her Scale for Assessment of Negative Symptoms (1983) and Scale for the Assessment of Positive Symptoms (1984).

Crow (1990)—in his two syndrome hypothesis of schizophrenia in 1980—described negative symptoms as relating to changes in brain structure, and positive symptoms as relating to biochemical change. The changes in structure were seen as occurring early. The positive symptoms were attributed to chemical changes and were associated with acute illness.

We recognize change in brain structure as occurring primarily in two ways: either by a partial return to an early developmental mind/brain, and/or by a partial fixation to an early mind/brain. In either case, the change in structure is secondary to activity; the higher cortical structures either partially atrophy because of disuse or partially fail to develop because of disuse—as the earlier structures of the brain either become or remain the dominant sites of activity.

In addition to the changes in brain structure caused by usage and dependent on emotional trauma, changes in brain development and structure can occur from early brain injury, or by chemical, viral, nutritional and emotional trauma in the second trimester, as referenced in *Second Trimester Factors* in Chapter One. It may also be affected by genetic influences.

The early changes, whether caused by early reactivation of infant fixation points, or determined by early physical, metabolic, chemical or viral injury, or by genetic factors—are thought to be irreversible, whereas later changes in structure, brought about by a later reactivation of the early trauma sites and disuse atrophy of higher cortical centers—may be reversible if not too long-standing.

Konrad Lorenz in 1973 shared a Nobel Prize in medicine for his work on imprinting (Kaplan and Saddock, 1994). He demonstrated that certain learning takes place only during brief but critical early stages of development. Pearce and Doman also identified age specific learning. Children who were stroked and massaged for the first 24 hours of life could run by age six months and kittens that were not licked on the abdomen immediately after birth had difficulty with locomotion (Pearce). Infants stimulated during the first two years with mathematical "dot" cards learned to do instant complex calculations in their heads that adults cannot do, and when trained with musical sounds they learned perfect pitch (Doman). The unique age specific learning abilities result from passing through the developmental brain, from the phylogenetically earliest structures to the most advanced. In the process, either the structures and their unique functions are activated and "turned on" or they are not. Once the infant has passed through that developmental area of the brain, it is no longer accessible for first time use.

This represents great conservatism of the structures of the brain: the new mammalian brain does not have to duplicate all the functions of the old mammalian brain, and the old mammalian brain does not have to duplicate all the functions of the reptilian brain. When properly sequentially activated, phylogenetically earlier structures/abilities are accessible and available for use later in life.

This passing through the early brain takes place in the first months and years of life. This early shift, from one region of the brain to the next, accounts for the reason why there are changes in brain structure when there is a return to or a fixation in an early traumatic experience/brain site. Traumas of later origin are not etched in the phylogenetically older regions of the brain. Already in the second and third year of life there is massive development in the language center, which is advanced well beyond all other species. When this area of the brain is developing, language "imprinting" is maximal. Reportedly young Berlitz was reared in a large multilingual family with each member instructed to speak to him in a different language, and by age four he was fluent in twelve languages.

Thus, during the earliest formative years we sequence through earlier brain structures, activating, developing and gaining access to them for later use. Early trauma sites become fixed "like epileptogenic focal points" which later can be reactivated "and caused to perseverate" (Paul MacLean, 1984, personal correspondence). The earliest sites are in the phylogenetically earliest parts of the brain—which produce proportionately greater amounts of important neuro-transmitters. When the earlier sites are reactivated, there is an increase in dopamine production in the midbrain and a relative decrease in activity in higher cortical centers. As higher functions (e.g., driving a car) are processed in accordance with earlier reality (e.g., the "everyone is watching me and following me wherever I go" reality of age 14 months), aberrant neuronal pathways develop in between, in the hippocampus.

To the extent that earlier sites remain active, there is less develop-ment of later sites. The precursors of schizophrenia and the negative signs are recognizable—as well as the reduced brain volume. These factors correspond with type II schizophrenia as described by Crow. Patients with type II schizophrenia are vulnerable to acute exacerba-tions later in life, however, and can then exhibit positive symptoms, biochemical change and further deterioration.

Patients who experience a trauma during infancy then appear to re-cover fully and develop normally only to have a sudden psychotic episode later in life, have a better prognosis—but they too can deterio-rate, regress totally, or fail to recover completely. We do not see a sharp boundary between type II and type I. It may be more of a continuum. Patients may carry forward from infancy *any* degree or amount of negative symptomatology or precursors of schizophrenia, and may or may not develop a psychosis later in life.

Delayed posttraumatic stress disorder of adult origin is similar in that one can see any gradation of bland denial or numbing prior to an acute incapacitating reaction. Or the person can have the excitatory symptoms of posttraumatic stress disorder and still move into a more incapacitating state when the posttraumatic stress disorder is more fully activated.

The bland denial and numbing of posttraumatic stress disorder from adulthood corresponds to the negative symptomatology that festers in type II schizophrenia from the time of the original trauma to the time of the first acute psychosis. The excitatory symptoms of adult PTSD corresponds with the wild and more chaotic positive symptoms found in type I schizophrenia. What we are observing are combinations and gradations of the two categories, as measured on continuums. For convenience, and in keeping with the concepts of identifying categories and separate distinct diagnostic entities, arti-ficial boundaries have been created. But it is all one process.

PHYLOGENETIC SHIFT TO TRAUMA OF EARLIER SPECIES:

In normal individuals, under extreme threat, we must not rule out a *phylogenetic* shift as well. In the author's personal study of Bernard Goetz, for example, there were eight or nine clear signals that he was about to be robbed. According to Goetz, however, it was not until the very last signal, when he saw the smile on the person's face and the gleam in his eye, that he went totally berserk. His mind raced back three years to the earlier time when thugs pulverized his kneecap and tried to throw him through a glass door. He returned so completely to that earlier point in time that even the famous statement "You look okay, here's another: *bang*" more likely came from the *fantasies* surrounding the first mugging. Survival behavior also ran deep enough that it is believed he tapped earlier resources in his brain. The human brain not only contains the new mammalian brain, but also includes the old mammalian brain and the reptilian brain as well (Paul MacLean, 1973, 1985). The entire animal kingdom has survival mechanisms built into it. Therefore, survival is built into the human species from much earlier times.

The entire question of how much time elapsed between the fourth and fifth shots was a moot point. After firing the last round, he wished he had more bullets to shoot them all again. Next, he thought about digging the first one's eyes out with his key. He then reached in his pocket and fumbled for his key. Up until this point, he was still in the survival mind/brain/reality mode of behavior, which dictates: "rip, tear, bite and claw until there is no sign of life left." **This is "built in" and need not come from one's own personal experience.** As Goetz reached in his pocket for his key, he noted a look of fear and submission in the first one's eyes. It was this look of submission which started to bring him out of his survival state. This also is a phenomenon that is "built in" and is related to earlier mammalian species. During the mating season when the losing animal shows a sign of submission, the victor stops attacking. In wolves, for example, the loser gives the winner a clear shot at his throat, and fighting ceases.

What brought Goetz completely out of the survival mode was the sight of a woman laying on the floor. His first thought was "My God, did I hit an innocent bystander?" His total concern for her at that point demonstrated clearly that he was out of the survival mind/brain/reality mode of behavior, as he was thinking about someone else's life instead of his own.

Based on Goetz' survival instinct/behavior, as well as what brought him out of the fight mode, it is postulated that a normal person may return not only to a trauma of earlier times in his own life, but in extreme cases he may reach more deeply into the phylogenetically older recesses of his brain to reactivate primordial trauma and survival mechanisms of earlier species.

Paul MacLean, in personal correspondence regarding "the Anatomy and Psychodynamics of Psychosis" (McKenzie, 1984), agreed with the author and wrote: "It seems quite reasonable that traumatic experiences in infancy and early childhood could set up a storm in those unstable structures of the phylogenetically old parts of the telencephalon that appear to be involved in the separation response. Somewhat analogous to an epileptogenic focus, the poorly damp-ened neural mechanisms would allow the storm to 'perseverate' or to be easily reactivated." This is the mechanism by which the authors believe the schizophrenic process operates. There are two areas of ac-tivity in the mind/brain of the schizophrenic: the adult and the re-awakened infant. When the functional reality of the reawakened infant portion of the mind/brain predominates, the result is acute psychosis. The same process or mechanism is thought to apply to all PTSD of the delayed type, where a small locus of activity of the mind/brain predominates. This is not a totally new concept. Janet (1894, 1897) observed "dissociated nuclei of consciousness" that were independent from the central personality and developed in re-sponse to traumatic events. With schizophrenia, we are looking at a very early nucleus of consciousness from long prior to rational adult memory, which is reawakened by a subsequent trauma and then continues to co-exist with adult mind/brain/reality.

7

Schizophrenia, PTSD, Autism, Symbiosis, Anorexia Nervosa, Alcohol and Drug Dependence

FURTHER COMPARISONS BETWEEN SCHIZOPHRENIA AND PTSD:

The mechanism that causes cognitive impairment in the schizophrenic may cause the cognitive impairment in the person with PTSD as well. If an earlier part of the mind/brain is activated and becomes a center of activity, it stands to reason that other areas by comparison are less active. When the schizophrenic is acutely ill, he may ruminate on two or three thoughts to the exclusion of all else. While this is extreme, all gradations are possible. Also, *those who are experiencing extreme PTSD and a return to a helpless state, may be returning partially to a helpless state during infancy,* but not as fully as the schizophrenic. Persons suffering from PTSD have elevated MMPI scores for depression (scale #2) and for schizophrenia (scale #8) (Wilson & Walker, 1990). This may represent a partial return to the mind/brain/reality of the first two years and ten months of life. Based on our findings of a return to age specific trauma during infancy, we predict that if Vietnam PTSD veterans were examined to compare elevated MMPI rating scale #2 and elevated MMPI rating scale #8 for incidence of sibling birth at various ages, the elevated schizophrenia scale would likely

61

correlate with increased sibling birth 9–18 months and the depression scale with increased incidence of sibling birth 24 to 34 months.

In September, 1993, the first author evaluated a 46 year old woman who exemplified this hypothesis for depression quite well. She was among 51 victims evaluated in Central America from the July 18, 1993 Sahsa Airline crash in Managua, Nicaragua. While she met full criteria for post-traumatic stress disorder, the horrible experience of the crash also awakened a trauma from her third year of life, and she became extremely depressed and suicidal. The intensity of the depression and self-blame clinically matched that of persons traumatized at two years two to three months, and when questioned, she revealed that she had a sibling two years three months younger. Her MMPI rating scale #2 would have been markedly elevated because she met the criteria for major depression, melancholic type.

The authors further predict that there will be an elevation of both the schizophrenia and the depression rating scales among persons with post-traumatic stress disorder who have siblings in the schizoaffective range, 18 to 24 months younger.

"Ex-post facto" considerations do not apply to a research design of this type because we are comparing the incidence of one early trauma at a particular age among persons with one condition to the incidence of the same trauma at the same age among persons with another condition. Furthermore, the birth of a sibling is recognized as a severe trauma to many infants whereas there is little difference to a child growing up whether the sibling is 17 or 19 months younger. The data is "hard data" because either there was or was not a sibling born during the specific age interval, and either there is or is not a designated elevation in the specific rating scale. The McKenzie research design was first described by Silva and Miele (1977), and detailed further by McKenzie (1986b). It is elaborated further in Section II of this book.

Measurements in complete populations will identify correlations between disease processes and ages of original trauma. Extreme guilt and self-condemnation, for example, may have a peak correlation with trauma at age two years two to three months. Precipitating stressors are also important in the two trauma mechanism, and eventually a relative hierarchy of precipitating trauma will be established for each illness. Each precipitating trauma can vary in intensity, and a mild trauma in the present can awaken an extreme trauma in the past, causing the infant trauma to be the more important factor, or an extreme trauma in the present can awaken a mild trauma in the past, causing the present trauma to be the more significant factor.

Thus, extreme actions that would cause maximum guilt, could awaken relatively milder but related traumas in the distant past. A population of veterans who were forced to commit horrible acts, for example, would likely reveal a higher elevation in the depression scale when compared to an overall PTSD population. This would not preclude a higher incidence of sibling birth at 25–34 months, however, among those who scored high on the depression scale. On a large enough scale, all factors, past and present, can be revealed and their relative significances determined.

Many scholars of PTSD have noted the relationship between PTSD and other serious emotional disorders. Van der Kolk (1988) identified "a remarkable parallel between protest and despair phases of an infant's response to parental separation and the hyperarousal and numbing states found in PTSD." Here he was noting the infant's response to what we consider the primary original trauma in schizophrenia, and he was comparing it to the adult's PTSD response to trauma later in life. The epitome of hyperarousal and numbing is seen in the two phases of catatonic schizophrenia, and interestingly enough, the excitatory phase in catatonic schizophrenia in one of the 300 schizophrenic patients studied appeared to demonstrate clinically the birth struggle. If birth ultimately is discovered to be the origin, then the extremes of catatonic schizophrenia should be expected—because birth represents the earliest trauma (and therefore the maximum vulnerability) and at the same time the maximal degree of protest-numbing (catatonic excitement vs. stupor) effect.

Krystal (1984) notes that traumatized adults often regress to stereotyped emotional and behavioral patterns including infantile dependency, obsessive compulsive behavior and difficulty modulating intensity of aggression. This is in keeping with a partial return to infancy. Beebe (1975) noted an increase in schizophrenia among those who experienced the most severe trauma. DeFazio (1978) noted that the contraction of ego function in PTSD can resemble the deterioration of ego function in schizophrenia. Van der Kolk (1989) notes the frequent elevation of scores of Johnston & Holtzman's (1979) thought disorder index among patients with PTSD, despite the absence of psychotic thinking. Kinzie & Boehnlein (1989) pointed out that just as depression and substance abuse can coexist with PTSD, so can schizophrenia-like symptoms. The present authors again emphasize, however, that the depression or "schizophrenia-like symptoms" may relate to the age-specific antecedent trauma that are present to be reawakened. Lifton & Olson (1976) point to the vulnerability to stress and the tendency to exacerbation in PTSD as being similar to the process in chronic schizophrenia. Doyle & Bauer (1989) describe attention deficit hyperactivity disorders and relate them in particular to early trauma of multiple out-of-home placements. The present authors note that babies are in constant motion, and hyperactivity in children is a partial return to an earlier, more active time. Janet (1893) observed that psychological trauma sometimes leads to a regression to earlier developmental stages. Again the authors maintain this depends on early trauma sites that were already present to be awakened. Gil et al. (1990) summarizes the literature illustrating cognitive deficits of PTSD and other emotional disorders, citing Chapman & Chapman (1973, 1978) and Archibald & Tuddaham (1965) for general correlates, Calev et al. (1983) for correlation with cognitive deficits of schizophrenia, and Calev & Erwin (1985) and Calev et al. (1986) for correlation with cognitive deficits of depression. Gil does not conclude there is a cognitive deficit specific to PTSD, and he suggests the deficits are likely a secondary consequence of general psychiatric symptomatology. The present authors relate this deficit to a movement in the direction of using earlier developmental portions of the brain, to a narrowing of the field of consciousness similar to that described by Janet in regard to hysteria (1909), and to the excessive mental energy utilized by the trauma sites and the repression of them. Janet (1893) notes the personality of the traumatized individual can no longer continue to enlarge by the addition or assimilation of new elements. It is as though the individual were attached to an unsurmountable obstacle. The authors believe this unsurmountable obstacle is the area of activity and repression pertaining to the particular trauma and to its reawakened earlier antecedents. The post-traumatic decline described by van der Kolk (1989), referencing Janet, runs a close parallel to the course and to the dementia that results from schizophrenia.

RELATIONSHIP BETWEEN SUBSTANCE DEPENDENCE & PTSD:

The increased incidence of alcohol and drug dependence among those with PTSD may also relate to the *two trauma* mechanism. McCormick et al. (1989), in pointing to the high incidence of drug and alcohol dependence in persons with PTSD, draws from his broad clinical experience to make the astute observation that PTSD patients suffer from all disorders of impulse control. This strengthens the argument for adult PTSD returning the person not only to the trauma in adult life, but to previous trauma at an earlier age when there was poor impulse control. When helplessness in the present links up with helplessness during infancy, any prolonged stress or frustration of infancy can be awakened and carry with it the desire to put something in the mouth to feel better.

EARLIER ONSET DELAYED PTSD FROM INFANCY:

McKenzie (1981) redefines serious emotional disorder as a coexistence of two minds in one skull: the adult mind and the reawakened mind—and brain—of the troubled infant. Thus, with the schizophrenic, the adult mind may be partially operating, but it may be under the control of and acting in accordance with the realities/needs/desires of an infant part of the mind. In *childhood* schizophrenia, since there was not as long a delay prior to onset of the illness, there is the coexistence of the child's mind and the reawakened mind and brain of the troubled infant. In *infantile autism*, since the onset occurs at the time of the trauma, with no period of delay, there is only the mind of the infant, combined with whatever the infant mind/brain is able to learn. (For a discussion of the neurological factors in autism, see section entitled Circumcision in Chapter 13.)

Symbiosis is a similar disorder. One interesting eight year old boy, who was evaluated by Bruno Bettelheim as well as by both authors, presented clinically as having symbiosis. A terrible trauma occurred at age 20 months, when the mother was raped in front of her husband and child. Following this experience, the mother became psychotic and thus, subsequent to the initial trauma, she was physically present but emotionally absent to the child during the remainder of his early formative years. As a result, his development, including his speech, was arrested at age 20 months. Had the woman recovered from her psychosis within a few days, her son might have returned to normal development, but then would have been vulnerable to the later development of schizo-affective range type of schizophrenia upon separation or rejection from some other "most important person" later in life.

DRUG AND ALCOHOL DEPENDENCE:

Alcohol and drug dependence include processes somewhat similar to those for schizophrenia and depression. The alcoholic may drink socially for twenty or thirty years, and then if there is a major separation or loss, he may find that he is unable to stop drinking. He may decide to have only one drink, but once he has that drink, he is no longer the same person who decided to have only one drink. He becomes the infant on the bottle and acts according to the infant on the bottle reality. He drinks until the belly is full and then passes out.

One question defied clinical explanation for 20 years: Why does the alcoholic, who *dreads* taking the first drink, take it nonetheless. He knows that it leads to the "binge" during which he may be mugged and break bones, will have terrifying DTs, develop pneumonia, or progress into liver failure and die. Ultimately the answer revealed itself: it is the *infant* who is cold, wet, hungry, teething and who cries for minutes and hours, which seem like days and weeks, until finally the mother comes along, picks him up, dries him off, holds him and feeds him. It is that *moment of bliss* which the alcohol dependent individual is trying to recapture, and he seeks this out when he begins to feel unhappy or lonely. He seeks something to put in his mouth that will make him feel good. An irony is that most often it facilitates his return to an age when he was very unhappy, and he becomes more depressed.

Clinically the alcohol dependent returns to an earlier part of the mind and brain. This was verified by one alcoholic who returned to visit a pub he frequented twelve years earlier, before he had attained sobriety. He had recalled this particular pub as being huge, palatial, filled with tables and chairs, and having a bar that extended out into infinity. When he returned, he was shocked to find that it was a small room with three small tables and a bar that was only twelve feet long. But to the one year old infant, who weighs 20 pounds instead of 200, the room appears ten times as large. This was also one of the early reality perceptions of Gary Heidnik while in his psychosis, because his plan was to house ten women and one hundred babies in a tiny basement of a row home in North Philadelphia. Only the infant brain can conceptualize the area as being that large. When an adult returns to visit the grammar school he once attended, he may be startled to find that the lockers which came to the top of his head are now at his belt line, and that the huge corridors are narrow little hallways. This is comparing reality of the child to the reality of the adult. The comparison of the infant to the adult is several times greater.

Recently a recovered schizophrenic woman described her first acute psychosis as beginning with the grocery store growing immense in size and sounds becoming much louder—as she moved into the infant mind/brain. Another schizophrenic woman had anorexia nervosa. She was a tall woman but weighed only 85 pounds. She reports that when she looked into the mirror during the height of her illness, she thought to herself "My God, I'm huge." And, of course, to a 23 pound baby, an 85 pound hulk is enormous. The infant part of her mind had intense needs for the mother and was kept highly activated by contact with any family member. By following a simple recommendation of separating from original family, she quickly returned from the infant reality and both the psychosis and the anorexia nervosa disappeared.

In addition to size and sound, time is distorted (Sharron, 1988), distances seem farther, and pain is experienced as being more intense. One patient regressed to age one year ten months in a general hospital setting because the nurses withheld or delayed medications. The withholding of medications returned her to a time when her mother withheld gratifications. Her pain was excruciating. When transferred to a psychiatric hospital the next week, the regression reversed, and *the same chronic pain that had been experienced as excruciating to the infant was experienced as relatively mild to the adult.*

Not only is time distored in schizophrenia, but it is distorted in normal individuals during extreme trauma. Among the 51 victims evaluated by the first author from the July 18, 1993 Sahsa Airline crash in Managua, Nicaragua, more than half of the victims estimated it took between five to ten minutes for the plane to come to a stop after it struck the ground—but in reality this could have taken only 30 to 40 seconds. The survivors of the June 22, 1994 Wings of Alaska Airline disaster, who also were evaluated by the first author, experienced their ordeal in frigid waters off Juneau as lasting up to five hours, whereas in actuality it was closer to one.

Origins of many serious emotional disorders are sometimes related to single experiences that are terrifying to the infant. Sometimes there are multiple trauma and sometimes the trauma occur at different stages of development. There may be precursors to the trauma causing the traumatic events to be more frightening, and there may be subsequent years of minor traumata (criticisms, rejections, failures) that cause the unconscious core nucleus of consciousness to magnify, augment and grow—even while remaining repressed and unconscious (See diagrams A–E).

The origin of drug and alcohol dependence was found to correlate with prolonged stress during infancy. In the former Russian satellite countries such as Lithuania, the women were paid to stay home with the babies for the first two months of life and then, between 2 months to 24 months, they were given reduced pay, such that most were forced to return to work. At 24 months, the women had no choice but to return to work. As a result, their babies' needs were not adequately met and they remained "infants on the bottle." For some, there is a continuous attempt at oral gratification from early childhood through adult life, while for others there is an awakening of those needs at a later time by stressors that are in some way similar to the first. It is interesting to note that Kraemer (1984) found that monkeys with early separation experiences are more susceptible to the abuse of alcohol. While it was not explored as to whether or not separation produced autism or set the stage for development of schizophrenia in this group of primates, it is clear that they returned to seeking oral gratification, and it is suspected that their early oral needs had not been met.

Hagan (1987) discovered that 83 percent of cocaine dependent women in one treatment center had parents who were cocaine or alcohol dependent. This is "*second* generation dependence." An intoxicated or drugged mother cannot attend as adequately to the needs of the baby, and when the needs of the infant—which are enormous—are not met, those needs may remain fixed, i.e., that area of the mind/brain/reality/behavior/feeling may remain more active and seek fulfillment forever. Often it becomes activated at a future time when other related needs are not met. It is likely that "*first* generation substance dependence" results from prolonged stress/maternal deprivation for reasons other than substance dependence which caused the second generation mother to be unavailable. In all fairness to the mothers of persons who become substance dependent—as with mothers of schizophrenics—the trauma during infancy need not necessarily have been great, because an extreme trauma in the present can return a person to a relatively milder trauma in the past. Schwartz (1989), in studying PTSD, also concluded that an extreme trauma in the present can overshadow the importance of antecedents.

NEED FOR THE MOTHER:

Not only does the infant want its needs met, but based on animal studies, the baby wants its needs met by its own mother. Harlow (1958) confirmed the need for the mother with his landmark study of primates. One hundred twenty million years of patterning of the mammalian brain has invested the infant with the desire to be with the mother and the mother to be with the infant. In the migration of the wildebeest across Africa, if the mother and infant separate while crossing a lake, they swim back and forth searching for one another until they drown. A mother seal is able to pass by 5,000 baby seals to find her very own, and neither she nor her baby has doubt as to whom they belong nor whom they want. Thus, the human infant likely prefers the mother, and the mother may be difficult to replace. Mother substitutes also fall short of the mark in another way: according to Spitz (1945), the mother is able to stimulate the infant more than any other person, and early stimulation, according to Doman (1984) and Pearce (1977, 1985) is crucial for mental growth and development.

8

Borderline Patients, Adolescents

BORDERLINE PATIENTS:

Separation in the first weeks or months of life could be the origin of borderline disorders, since borderline individuals have an exceedingly high rate of adoption. In 1984, at the Institute for Living in Hartford, it was observed that 25 percent of their borderline patient population had been adopted. At Élan One in Maine, a boarding school/treatment center which accepts troubled adolescents who are not schizophrenic, G.E. Davidson (1985) reported that 35 percent, or 56, of their 160 clients were adopted. A large portion of these children were borderline, but the population included other personality disorders, conduct disorders, identity, impulse and substance abuse disorders. According to Davidson, nearly all the adoptions took place in the first two weeks of life. In a cross-sectional survey of 15,416 children throughout the United States, Zill (1985) determined that two percent of the overall population were adopted. This means that of the 160 children at Élan One, only three should have been adopted instead of 56. This is like flipping a coin 59 times and having it come up heads 56. Using the binomial theorem, this would happen approximately once in one trillion trials. Since the adopteds at Elan One were mostly adopted in the first two weeks of life, this demonstrates a correlation between severely disturbed non-psychotic children and trauma occurring in the first month of life. While other factors may differ in the lives of adopteds, separation from the biological mother had already

71

been identified as the primary infant trauma that leads to serious emotional disorders.

Recently, a man, who had been borderline all his life, suddenly at age 60 decided that he simply wanted to lie in bed or eat. When he was hungry, he ate and then took a nap, and then later he would get up and eat, and then go back to bed. More noteworthy is the fact that to him this was perfectly normal behavior, which indicated that it originated at a time when it *was* normal, i.e. it was the behavior of the *newborn* who simply feeds and sleeps. Also of note is the fact that this man, throughout his life, had been extremely obsessive compulsive and stored away everything, just like an animal of an earlier species—such as a rodent. If he managed to go to McDonald's for a hamburger, the wrapper was folded into a precise little square and placed inside the box, and the box was saved and stacked with 100 or more identical boxes from the same restaurant. Every newspaper and every magazine was similarly saved, until there was no room left in the house.

This person was traumatized in the first month of life. His compulsive behavior called to mind that of a woman who was traumatized at age seven days when she lay dying of septicemia, in a pediatrics ward, separated from her mother. Throughout her early childhood, she continued to force her mother to play a game with her in which the mother would leave but would sneak back in through the window. The thrust of the game was that the mother really did not go away (as she had been forced to when her baby was in the hospital). In adult life, although the woman achieved high academic degrees, she remained infantile and sometimes called her mother on the telephone, insisting that she and her mother leave the phones off the hook throughout the night. Symbolically, this provided the umbilical connection that existed just prior to the original trauma. This woman also exhibited extreme obsessive compulsive symptoms. At times she would ruminate over the meaning of a word until she reached a frenzy, searching through dictionaries and encyclopedias to find the exact meaning, which was never quite right. This behavior was so intense when it occurred that it matched only the primitive behavior observed in a Japanese beetle, trapped in a glass jar. The beetle raced frantically around the jar, continuing on the same path, for hours. Clinically, the two behaviors were in some way similar.

Borderline states frequently appear to correlate with the earliest trauma. Mahler (Masterson) attributes the early trauma to separation and loss during the separation–individuation phase of development, and especially during the rapprochement subphase, between

16 and 24 months. This age of origin is a possibility, because many symptoms of borderline personality disorder match symptoms of the 18–24 month age range. We still hold the opinion that the origin could be in the first months of life and we eagerly await the survey results. This could end speculation. If the borderline syndrome is related to early trauma, the peak age of origin and the age range of origin will surface quickly, along with the nature and duration of the original trauma.

Obsessive compulsive behavior frequently accompanies borderline personality disorder. Phylogenetically earlier regions of the brain may be the first called into action, and extreme, frantic obsessive compulsive behavior found in some borderline individuals may resemble that of the most primitive members of the Animal Kingdom. Anatomically, severe obsessive compulsive symptoms correlate with increased activity in phylogenetic older structures of the brain, especially the cingulate gyrus, the head of the caudate nucleus, and the orbital cortex (predominantly on the left). The shift to anatomically earlier structures of the brain supports the possibility of early infant origin. According to Baxter (1994) recovery results in the normalization of glucose metabolism in the caudate, which further supports our concept of the shift in areas of brain activity during the disease process, and a return to the prior area of activity as recovery takes place.

A marked increase in incidence of incest has been noted among borderline individuals (Kernberg, O., 1975), which would seem to implicate trauma of later origin. The increased incidence of incest among borderline individuals, however, in part may be a *result* of the disease process, just as the "schizophrenogenic mother" usually is a result of the patient's shift to the infant mind, rather than being the cause of the disease process. The increased incidence of incest could in part relate to the increased number of adopteds among the borderline population and the fact that biologically, with adopteds, it is not incest. Careful studies ultimately will reveal which correlations are causative in nature.

ADOLESCENCE:

During normal adolescence there is a recapitulation of the original separation–individuation phase (Pearson, 1958), which begins in the forth or fifth month of life and ends by age 36 months. Since the new struggle for independence is similar to the earlier one, it reawakens, to some extent, an earlier part of the mind. This leaves the young teenager more vulnerable to a return to the earlier mind/brain/reality.

At the earlier age, when the whole world was the mother, criticism or disapproval was like a dagger in the heart. With the early wounds partially awakened, helpful suggestions and friendly advice are vehemently defended against in that they resemble criticism and are perceived as such—particularly if the advice comes from parents. Pathological diagnoses often are reserved until after the person is beyond this tumultuous stage, as the partial awakening of the earlier mind/brain/feeling can resemble all facets of serious mental disorders.

Having referred to adolescence as a tumultuous stage of development, we feel obliged to address current analytical thinking: According to Garfinkel (1992), most analysts now regard adolescence as a period of quiescence. The onset of adult illnesses and the increased suicide rate would seem to indicate otherwise, however. Dementia praecox, the former term for schizophrenia, literally means dementia beginning at puberty. Puberty remains an important age of onset for schizophrenia. Major depression, OCD and other adult psychiatric disorders begin in adolescence, and the suicide rate increases dramatically. Thus we opt for the opinion written in ancient hieroglyphics on the walls of the tombs in Egypt, 5,000 years ago, exclaiming: "What's going to happen to the world as a result of the way teenagers are today?"

9

Further Comparisons with Delayed PTSD. Perpetuating Factors in all Forms of PTSD

COMPARISON OF DELAYED TYPE PTSD FROM ADULT EXPERIENCE AND DELAYED TYPE PTSD FROM INFANCY:

Examples in the Adult:

In a recent account (Samuel, 1990) one Veteran returned from Vietnam and functioned relatively well for the next 15 years. He was decorated with three purple hearts, but his most terrifying experience in Vietnam was when his company accidentally disturbed a large number of hornets. They were totally defenseless as hundreds of thousands attacked. Some men had hundreds of stingers embedded in their face. When this Veteran returned from Nam, he married, was gainfully employed and raised a family. His life was a success until one day, at his place of employment, he found the ceiling of the men's room covered with hornets. His life suddenly became a living nightmare as he was no longer able to work, sleep or function.

In another veteran, the carefully studied case of "Mr. D." reported by van der Kolk and Ducey (1984, 1989), Rorschachs were administered before and after the original trauma was awakened. "Card after card reflected the same shift from earlier bland denial to later excruciating living of past horrors...." The earlier experiences, which had sealed over, were awakened 10 years later by three traumatic experiences as a police officer.

One of the authors' patients had a similar experience with a 44 year delay. In combat training in 1945 he had experienced extreme panic because he was not fully recovered from meningitis. This led to angioneurotic edema and a near death experience. Forty-four years later he was in a car accident. When he was given an MRI, the instructions "don't move," combined with the repetitive clicking sound, caused him to hallucinate tracer bullets flying overhead, which he saw with his eyes closed and open. There was a return of the same anxiety state, the angioneurotic edema, and the nightmares throughout each night.

Examples of Delayed PTSD From Infancy:

Many examples have already been given. The mechanism is the same. The precipitating trauma for the *initial* acute illness or psychosis, however, is always a major loss, separation or rejection from an important person or group, whether real, imagined, anticipated or implied. This is because trauma to the infant, almost without exception, involves a relative degree of physical or emotional separation from the mother. Sometimes the original stressor is augmented by physical pain, illness or previous trauma, but fear of separation from the main caregiver—regardless how brief—is the primary factor.

The higher incidence of psychosis in PTSD among Cambodian refugees, as reported by Kinzie & Boehnlein (1989), in part may relate to an increase in frequency of the major stressor of losing important loved ones in the present. Such a severe loss as watching loved ones executed in the present could awaken even some of the relatively milder threats of separation during infancy, resulting in a return to the infant mind nonetheless.

The Neuroses, PTSD & Delayed PTSD From Infancy:

The neuroses, as described by Freud, have been studied in depth, perhaps more than the psychoses and the PTSDs. Furthermore, the neurotic mechanism may be similar to the mechanism for posttraumatic stress disorder and delayed PTSD from infancy. Freud (1894) initially endorsed childhood trauma as the origin of many neuroses. Eventually he attributed the neuroses to fantasies of childhood. The authors believe it is both, and that even a small trauma can grow into an enormous fantasy. Fantasies must have some basis in reality, yet what they are based on is not as extreme as what the person eventually comes to experience. A child is frightened by a parent, for example, and has nightmares about monsters or witches that far exceed the power or evil intent of the parent. A child who observes nudity may dream several years later of a sea serpent 100 yards long. Thus the content of the nucleus of consciousness expands in terms of the items it contains. With the neuroses, with PTSD from adulthood and with PTSD from infancy, the authors believe the isolated nuclei of consciousness are not static; they grow, like abscesses of the mind. Every dream, every memory, every flashback (conscious *and unconscious*) may feed into the isolated nucleus of consciousness. Unconscious flashbacks may be more frequent than conscious flashbacks, and they may explain a portion of physiological "remembering." One eight year old girl, for example, came in for evaluation after being treated for a seizure disorder for more than one year following a car accident. It was discovered during the first interview that the "seizure disorder" occurred only during a certain TV program. Careful history revealed that the program began each day at 4:00 PM, and the car accident had occurred shortly after 4:00 PM. The "seizure" activity changed after interpretation, demonstrating a mental component to the physiological response. This type of mental activity increases the size of the core nucleus of consciousness. Fears, fantasies and dreams also cause it to expand. Each time the trauma is awakened—consciously or unconsciously—the defenses are called into play, and this-strengthens the defenses. Thus, as the core nucleus of consciousness abscess of the mind grows, the defensive wall thickens. Finally, when an experience outside the wall is sufficiently *intense and similar* to that which is inside the wall, the defensive barrier breaks down. Acute stresses such as associated with marriage, graduation, or becoming a parent, awaken earlier stresses and fantasies and precipitate the neuroses. A traumatic event can awaken childhood fears/fantasies and precipitate a phobia. A car backfiring will return a veteran to the front lines and combat readiness. Dire life circumstances can awaken prolonged stress during infancy and cause a person to return to the infant-on-the-bottle reality/needs/gratification (alcohol dependence), and the loss of a spouse can return one to the "loss" (fear of separation) from the earlier "most important person" during infancy, and bring about a *partial* return to the particular earlier mind/brain/reality/feeling/behavior/needs/desires/gratifications/chemistry/physiology and neuroanatomical sites that existed and were active at the precise earlier moment of the first trauma (schizophrenia and depression).

ONCE THE EARLIER MIND/BRAIN/REALITY IS ACTIVATED, IT REQUIRES VERY LITTLE TO KEEP IT ACTIVE:

The alcoholic need take only one drink.

"Mr. D." became upset by just looking at a Rorschach card after his PTSD had been activated (van der Kolk and Ducey, 1989).

Anxiety and panic attacks continue easily once the process is started.

The former Diagnostic and Statistical Manual of Mental Disorders (*DSM III*, American Psychiatric Association, 1980), notes that "Frequently an episode of Major Affective Disorder follows a psychosocial stressor...however, subsequent episodes may occur apparently without precipitating factors."

The word "apparently" was well chosen. The authors have found that both depression and schizophrenia, once precipitated or awakened by psychosocial factors, are easily *re*awakened or perpetuated by contact with persons who were present at the time of the initial trauma during infancy, i.e., members of the original nuclear family. It is family contact that serves most often as the precipitating factor for subsequent acute illnesses.

Bruno Bettelheim (personal correspondence, Oct. 1986) concurred with this finding among schizophrenic children and noted the "pernicious impact which contact with parents or other close relatives can have." G.W. Brown (1966, 1970) was commissioned by the Medical Research Council of England to find what factors in the post mental hospital environment led to rehospitalization. One factor prevailed; those who returned to original family, versus living anywhere else, required more hospitalization. McKenzie (1981) identified this phenomenon as the "the trap of schizophrenia." Beginning with the first psychotic episode, the parent-child relationship becomes a parent-infant one. Thus when the patient is with the parent he *is* the infant, and the infant will never leave the parent. From the other direction, for the parent to separate becomes tantamount to giving up a baby. Both cling tenaciously therefore to the relationship that locks the patient into the infant mind/brain/reality, and each interaction reinforces the infant from both directions, thereby perpetuating the schizophrenic condition.

Since both schizophrenia and depression consist of the coexistence of the adult and the reawakened infant mind, and since the re-awakened infant mind has great needs of the family member, any contact whatsoever activates the infant mind and brain. Likewise, since drug and alcohol dependent individuals also return to infancy, their conditions and processes are kept active by contact with original family too. The needs of the reawakened infant mind become activated and seek oral gratification when in contact with the infant's original caregivers and other family members. Thus, a substance dependent person has to abstain from the substance *and* from the original family.

In conclusion, nearly all emotional disorders seem to relate meaningfully to this PTSD model: there is an initial trauma—either single or sometimes multiple—which can continue to grow. The original stressor may be brief or prolonged. There can be immediate and persistent illness or a delayed type response. When the traumatic experience is walled off as an abscess of the mind, internal and external stimuli can feed into it and cause it to grow, and as it increases in size, the defensive wall thickens. When a later trauma is *sufficiently similar and intense* to the first, the earlier experience/gestalt is activated and the person draws upon the earlier mind/brain/reality to cope with the later trauma. This may be accompanied by any mental, emotional, biochemical or physiological feature that existed at the earlier time. Once this earlier state is activated by a significant trauma in the present, very little is required to *re*activate or perpetuate it.

Age specific origins of various emotional disorders have been identified through cumulative observations over the 25 year period. By carefully applying the research design developed by McKenzie (Silva & Miele, 1977; McKenzie, 1986b), it may be possible to identify the specific age of origin of each symptom or emotional disorder that is related to early trauma. The authors have no attachment to any particular result, but are very interested to have this important developmental research carried out soon and with great care.

SUMMARY OF SECTION I:

The authors have identified a two trauma survival mechanism that appears to be a causal factor for several serious emotional disorders, including schizophrenia, depression, and substance dependence. The mechanism appears to be the same mechanism operating in all delayed type PTSD. Based on 25 years of cumulative histories and clinical observations, the authors have identified retrospectively the critical ages of original trauma for various categories of schizophrenia and depression and have identified the nature of the original traumas. As a result of identifying the nature of the original trauma and the age at which it occurs, the authors have provided a basis for prevention and for future prospective study.

II

RESEARCH

——10——

Research Design, Pilot Studies

Matters of statistics are best determined by statisticians, and for that reason the McKenzie research design was subjected to the scrutiny of a noted statistics scholar, Professor John deCani, former Rhodes Scholar, Chairman of the Department of Statistics at the University of Pennsylvania's Wharton Business School, and author of a textbook on statistics. Professor deCani endorsed the research design and the statistical analysis of the pilot study data. It is necessary to be clear on the validity of the research design and method because often a professional in one field presumes expertise in the area of statistics and tosses out a word such as "scatter distribution" or "ex post facto" as a means of dismissing findings about which he has doubt. This design is simple and it does its job.

By utilizing the revolutionary method and design, it is possible for the first time to establish which symptoms or disorders are related or are not related to infant trauma. It is also possible to identify the most likely mathematical peak age of origin and the age range of origin of each disorder or symptom related to infant trauma. Either the symptom or disorder correlates with a higher incidence of "hard data" known accidental occurrences at a specific age in months during infancy or it does not, and either it is significant or it is not.

J. Martin Myers, Chairman of the Department of Psychiatry at the Institute of the Pennsylvania Hospital for 29 years, recognized the merits of the research design and wrote in April, 1984, that the "ideas should be researchable—e.g., the prevalence of sibling births as a significant factor in the later development of schizophrenia when it occurs in the first 18 months period of life." He encouraged the research and wrote that "many of your thoughts, if validated, would help us greatly in understanding the development and treatment of schizophrenia."

The design is simple and yet profound. It reveals the significance of correlations between infant trauma and the later development of serious mental disorders, quickly and easily. If symptoms are related to early trauma, it reveals that, and if they are unrelated, it reveals that as well.

HERE IS HOW IT WORKS:

One known early infant trauma is selected, such as birth of a sibling, for example. Fifty years later it is known how many days old the first child was when the second was born, because birth dates are recorded. Birth of a sibling is a very traumatic experience to many infants/toddlers, and many researchers of infant psychology, including Margaret Mahler (1979), reported this to be a serious trauma. It is also "hard data": Either there was a sibling born or there was not. Ten researchers viewing the same data would concur.

For a simple pilot study, to determine if mental illness correlates with an increased incidence of infant trauma, we prefer the diagnostic category of "sick enough to be in a halfway house." This represents hard data; either they are in a halfway house for the mentally ill or they are not, and any number of researchers would agree—whereas ten experts might not agree on a particular diagnostic category. Most, but not all, of the subjects have schizophrenia. This means our data is less significant because we do not have a "pure culture" of schizophrenia. But an error in the direction of diluting the concentration of schizophrenics does not affect adversely the **validity** of the findings—i.e., if we can dilute the concentration of schizophrenics and still achieve statistical significance, then the results are even more valid.

Now we take a group of normal controls. These are 40 years and older because schizophrenia is unlikely to occur after that age. We could do Rorschachs on them and take detailed histories to screen out anyone with schizophrenic tendencies/features/symptoms/characteristics/histories. But once more we keep it loose so we do not get a "perfect" sample of super normal individuals. In other words, we again err in the direction of making the data less significant so as to not destroy the validity of the findings. We are still looking for a healthy group, however, and not simply the average individual. We want to compare the few percent who are most sick with the few percent who are the most well. If there is no correlation between early infant trauma and wellness vs. sickness, then there should be no significant difference in incidence of early trauma from one extreme end of the bell curve to the next.

For our first pilot study in 1985, we used a complete population of two halfway houses (N = 60). One question was asked: What was their age at the birth of the next sibling? Here we needed two birth dates: the patient's and that of the next sibling. Proprietors of the halfway houses gathered the data and we were not able to verify the accuracy of their data, but the data was consistent with findings from the cumulative histories of disturbed patients over the 25 year interval.

Next the first author polled the first 60 persons he encountered who had a full range of emotion and were leading useful productive lives—and for whom the author had no prior knowledge of sibling relationships. These individuals were then questioned as to their birth dates and date of birth of the next sibling.

From the two groups, there were 20 of the 120 individuals who had siblings born in the first 18 months of life.

Note that the design **concentrates** the data; instead of studying 120 individuals, we now studied 20 who had been traumatized between nine and eighteen months of age.

Like the flip of a coin, if early trauma between ages nine and eighteen months has no bearing on the later development of schizophrenia, then approximately ten should come from each group.

But 17 came from the "schizophrenic" group and three from the "super normal." This is like flipping a coin 20 times and having it come up heads 17. According to the binomial theorem, this should occur once in 1,000 trials. The data was significant. The pilot study showed a correlation between serious mental illness and an accidental traumatic experience that occurred between nine and eighteen months of age.

The looseness of the design was in the direction that would not detract from the validity. The total cost in man hours was approximately ten. To the extent it can be repeated, this simple study may do as much to establish the *origin* of serious mental disorders as the billions spent in biological research. This does not detract in any way from the importance of the very remarkable findings in terms of changes in biochemistry, physiology, neurosynapses, areas of activity in the brain, changes in the structure of the brain, etc. The importance of each finding stands on its own, and these factors must be studied because it is possible to interrupt the schizophrenic process at many levels—just as a chain can be broken at any link. But the correlation the McKenzie method makes is with an accidental occurrence that takes place prior to the identification of biololgical correlations, and prior to the recognized early precursors of schizophrenia. Since the trauma occurs before a biological change is identified, and because the traumatic experience is accidental and occurs long before the onset of the disease, it is clear that the traumatic experience can not be the *result* of the disease process. The same can not be said for any of the biological correlations. This sets this group of correlations totally apart from the biological ones, for biological change can be the result of the disease process.

Furthermore, the proof of the causal relationships is the fact that the schizophrenic or depressed patient returns to the age specific feelings/reality/behavior of the time/age of the original trauma, and the age of the original trauma can be estimated with accuracy prior to confirmation from history, based on the specific feelings/behavior/reality the patient is experiencing.

This is more apparent when we examine delayed post-traumatic stress disorder of later origin, such as from war trauma. When an explosion occurs next to a combat veteran and he flashes back to the earlier experience, we do not speak in terms of correlations between taking defensive action and having had earlier war experience. We make a direct inference that the veteran had a flashback to an earlier war trauma, and that his mini psychosis is caused by a sound in the present returning him to the particular age/time of a similar sound in the past, and that he returns to the same gestalt/mindset/reality/combat readiness and physiological response that accompanied the original trauma—even if the trauma had occurred 25 years earlier. This same reasoning should apply to schizophrenia. The original trauma has been identified, and upon a similar trauma of separation later in life the person "flashes back" to the earlier mind/brain/reality/feelings/behavior/chemistry/physiology and neuroanatomical site. **Every piece of disturbed reality and behavior in the schizophrenic matches in some way the reality and behavior of the infant at the specific time/age traumatized.** Thus our finding is not just a correlation. Biological correlations, aside from possible genetic predispositions, have not yielded evidence of being causally related, such as have the accidental traumatic experiences at specific ages during infancy.

1994 RESEARCH SURVEY:

In January, 1994, a new research design was introduced. Persons with schizophrenia and major depression were surveyed to determine their age at the birth of siblings who were less than three years younger. Many who met the *DSM-III-R* criteria for schizophrenia were in what we call the schizoaffective range. We included these individuals in the 1994 study and expanded the age range to 24 months.

Our hypothesis was that persons with schizophrenia, and persons with major depression who had a history of auditory hallucinations, would have a preponderance of siblings born between 12 and 24 months as opposed to 24 to 36 months, and persons with major depression who never heard voices would have a preponderance of sibling births 24 to 36 months as opposed to 12 to 24 months. In the general population the number of siblings born 12 to 24 months is very close to the number born 24 to 36 months, but the schizophrenic population had more than 75% of the siblings in the 12 to 24 month as opposed to the 24–36 month time interval. Every aspect of the study was significant beyond the .001 level.

More data is desired to pinpoint the peak age of origin and age range of origin for each symptom/diagnostic category, but the broad categories have already been identified beyond the .001 level of statistical significance.

To research a new finding in an established field is a special challenge. The weight of the evidence is against the researcher and proof is demanded before research grants are provided. Furthermore, this particular area of investigation does not advance the interests of pharmaceutical companies; it may be viewed as a threat to biological research—in which the universities are highly funded and invested; and it immediately offends patient and family groups because it does not single out a biological cause on which to pin the blame. Thus the progress in this 25 year effort has been hampered and delayed because it stands apart from current areas of research, and it does not augment or support commercial, academic or political interests in the field.

The research is in progress and the data will be forthcoming nonetheless. Information is being accumulated slowly. The design is simple and since it now is set forth, any careful researcher can begin making determinations. We encourage communication and coordination of research efforts so we may help identify and avoid pitfalls and so the data gathered may become cumulative from one study to the next. Presently we are acting as a central clearing house for data pertaining to infant trauma that correlates with serious mental disorders.

We have no attachments to any particular results. NONE. If subsequent research were to prove that there are no correlations between infant trauma and the later development of serious emotional disorders, then GREAT; we can eliminate a whole category of possible causes and search for something else! But meanwhile, prior to proof to the contrary, we would not endorse traumatic separations from the mother for infants/toddlers, nor would we recommend rearing a baby with a terry cloth surrogate mother holding a bottle—even if with modern day robotics it can change a diaper too.

SUBSEQUENT RESEARCH:

The 1985 pilot study was loose in the direction that would make the data less significant and thereby not detract from validity. Its only purpose was to determine if statistical analysis of actual data confirmed or negated impressions based on cumulative observations. It confirmed those findings.

The January 1994 study demonstrated beyond the .001 that schizophrenia was related to a traumatic event prior to age 24 months, that major depression with auditory hallucinations was related to emotional trauma prior to 24 months, and major depression without auditory hallucinations was related to emotional trauma between 24 and 36 months. It also demonstrated that the symptom of auditory hallucinations was produced by an emotional trauma prior to 24 months, or prior to the development of language and the massive development of the left posterior superior temporal gyrus. Sarnoff Mednick kindly put this to the test for us, using the Finnish database on 6,000 schizophrenic patients, revealing a very high level of statistical significance and confirming a substantially higher rate of schizophrenia among those with siblings less than two years younger.

All these findings represent gross general categories. Subsequent studies must do more. Each symptom and each disorder needs to be studied for correlations with early trauma. It is important to determine the most likely mathematical peak age and age range of origin for each symptom/disorder, and the relative degree of importance of each trauma. For example, clinically the age of origin of the most rigid inflexible paranoid schizophrenia is approximately 14 months, and the range appears to be 13 to 15 months. Paranoid schizophrenia extends beyond that range, but the rigid, inflexible quality with flattened affect (a *DSM-IV* exclusion) and the concept of the external "influencing machine" (Tausk, 1933, for example), seem to be features related to this age. Paranoid schizophrenia of age 17 months origin may be "people on TV are talking about me," and paranoid ideation that stems from the early portion (19–21 months) of the schizo-affective range is still less untenable: "people are talking about me." (These are cumulative impressions, not yet put to the test.)

If we were to use the parameter of age at birth of a sibling on 100 of the rigid paranoid schizophrenic patients, and compare them to age at birth of a sibling among 100 super normal individuals—to first check for validity—and then check the distribution of ages at birth of the next sibling among the patient population, we would find that the patients with the one diagnosis would cluster around one particular month, and there would be a mathematical most likely peak age of origin. This data could be cumulative and the peak age would shift slightly as more data was acquired. Among the first 10,000 matched pairs of paranoid schizophrenics and super normals, there would be a certain number of paranoid schizophrenics with siblings born at the peak age of vulnerability for paranoid schizophrenia, and there would be a much smaller number of super normal individuals with siblings born at that same particular peak age. Among the same group of paranoid schizophrenics and super normals, there would also be a certain number of individuals who suffered a sudden unexpected death of a father at the same age, or the sudden unexpected death of a mother at the same age. *Statistical analysis of the data would enable us to determine which is more traumatic at that particular peak age: the death of a parent or the birth of a sibling.* In the same way we can study documented moves to a new house or documented hospitalizations of the mother or the patient as a baby. In other words, *eventually we can determine the relative degree of trauma for the average of each particular type of experience.* This, of course, is extremely important for prevention, and of all the current research in psychiatry, this may be the most urgently needed.

──11──

Other Parameters for Study, Depression, Adoption

TIME OF YEAR RESEARCH:

Most are aware of the increased incidence of schizophrenia among those born late winter and early spring. Emotional disturbances and hospitalizations are also known to occur more during the holidays. This means that there is an increased incidence of mothers with young babies who became upset up and who have to be hospitalized during the holidays—which produces more traumatic separations at those times. Babies who are born in February are approximately ten months old at the next Hanukkah/Christmas or New Years, and they are approximately 22 months of age when it comes around again. Thus, one consideration for possible cause of the increased incidence of schizophrenia in late winter/early spring is the increase in traumatic separations during the holiday season combined with a peak age of vulnerability for schizophrenia.

This trauma factor could only represent a portion of the seasonal trauma, because in the southern hemisphere a similar seasonal pattern is reported, but their summer is our winter. Therefore, seasonal affective disorders may also account for the slight increase in schizophrenia among those born late winter/early spring in both hemispheres. Part of what may be regarded as seasonal affective disorder, however, may relate more to holidays, because some disturbed patients get sick whenever they attend annual family gatherings. If the process is mostly related to seasonal factors and not holiday gatherings, then viral etiologies or seasonal affective disorder in the mothers may play a more important role in this slight increase. This is discussed in Chapter One under the heading of Second Trimester Factors. All these factors deserve study, regardless if they account for only a small increase in schizophrenia. Even the smallest clue can lead to important findings.

PEAK AGE OF VULNERABILITY:

While seasonal factors might not be important because they relate to only a very small percentage of the schizophrenic population (5–10%), the peak age of vulnerability and the overall distribution and age range of vulnerability are of vital importance and deserve intensive study. Here the birth of a sibling data is not helpful, because it allows only for the study of trauma after age nine months.

The sudden unexpected death of a parent, however, would be extremely useful (the impact of the sudden unexpected death of the father vs. the mother should be studied separately and together). Even though there are additional developmental factors related to being reared without one parent, the moment of loss is very traumatic. This is based on cumulative clinical observations as they correlate with expected age of trauma. This parameter will reveal the peak age of vulnerability for schizophrenia. We have very little data prior to ten months because of the lack of sibling births prior to that age. Likely the incidence of schizophrenia is higher with trauma after that age simply because of the fact that birth of a sibling is a frequent and severe trauma and can not occur until after that age. But it is possible that the infant could be more **vulnerable** to trauma at age eight months when he experiences stranger anxiety, for example. We do not yet know. Likely we will learn the age of origin of some of the more unusual disorders, such as the former diagnostic category of hebephrenia, which may be the peak age for ego-splitting—and which may coincide with the age of origin of multiple personality disorders. Age eight months is a possibility. This entire area is fertile for discovery.

In 1991 we encountered only one patient whose trauma definitely could be established as occurring at age six months—when the mother suddenly had to care for an older child who became ill. The patient's symptoms matched those of hospitalism or anaclitic depression. He was not delusional, but all emotion was gone and he was totally empty as he stared blankly ahead and said: "This is not me." Soon he even could not leave his apartment or feed himself. (Of interest is the fact that the 60 year old woman described under the heading of Inescapable Shock in Chapter 3, who was being chewed by a rat at age six months, did not experience a loss of her mother and did not show any signs of "hospitalism," but she returned precisely to the mental solution/response of the earlier time when she thought about trauma 60 years later.)

What is needed, on a large scale, is for psychiatrists from across the nation to determine the birth date of the patient and the date of the sudden, unexpected death of the mother, or father, of all their patients who lost a parent in the first three years of life, and to further make a diagnosis and a list of symptoms to send to our national registrar. Presently we are accepting and recording all such data. (Data related to symptoms and age at birth of a sibling is also welcomed.) Based on 25 years of cumulative observations, we expect the various disease categories to line up according to age of trauma. If there is a peak age of vulnerability for schizophrenia, random, unexpected deaths of parents should produce more schizophrenia at that age, the only presumption being a fairly uniform distribution of sudden accidental parental deaths over the first three years of life of the infant.

The same data would reveal the age of origin of all symptoms and disease categories related to trauma, the age of origin of borderline syndromes if related to trauma, and the age of origin of the more unusual types of schizophrenia. The data also would delineate the early cut off point for the age of origin of schizophrenia if one exists.

OTHER TRAUMAS TO STUDY, AND A POSSIBLE SHIFT FROM PREPONDERANCE OF ONE TRAUMA TO PREPONDERANCE OF ANOTHER:

While studying infant trauma, we are confronted with a number of factors that apply to normal and schizophrenic populations alike. The birth of a sibling is so traumatic to many infants that when it occurs it almost invariably outweighs other factors and registers as the significant trauma. But there may be a shift taking place in regard to infant trauma. Whereas the birth of a sibling represented approximately one-third of infant trauma, other traumas are becoming more frequent: more parents are separating and divorcing, and this is very traumatic to the infant. More mothers work and more than 50 percent of mothers with one year old babies now place them in daycare (Stains, 1987). Thus, there are more trauma to dilute the ones we study, and it is possible that the birth of a sibling, in future generations, will no longer represent the same percentage of infant trauma.

It will be important to search the early history for other traumas and to determine the relative impact of each early trauma on the infant at each age. Birth and death records are kept. Other records are harder to trace, such as when parents separate, when the mother starts work, when the family moves to a new apartment, or when the child starts daycare. Whenever the child or mother is hospitalized, this is recorded in hospital records and can serve to pinpoint the age of early trauma. In divorce, certificates are recorded, but this is not a fixed point of trauma because it is preceded by traumatic separations at varying intervals. Other factors must be considered when taking a detailed background history for early trauma—such as whether the patient is a twin or whether the patient is adopted. These are obvious areas for study. The birth of a sibling is not the only trauma that needs to be studied. Other early traumas need to be evaluated and the results compared to develop a relative severity for each trauma at each age. This is crucial for prevention. The trauma to prevent at age 12 months may be different from the trauma to prevent at age 20 months. Maybe the child can tolerate a move to a new house at age 26 months, but not at age 12 months—or vice versa. These are important determinations that must be made for preventive purposes.

While validity studies, related to simple, hard data parameters of known dates of origin are relatively simple to conduct, the overall project of determining the relative average degree of trauma for each traumatic event, including the ones that can not be dated precisely, will be a far more arduous task.

DEPRESSION STUDY:

In a complete population of 26 depressed individuals, *all* those who had siblings born 18-1/2 to 22 months younger (N = 4) heard voices, and *none* of those who had siblings born 24 to 34 months younger (N = 4) heard voices. The mutual exclusivity of this small sample population is significant beyond the .01 level. The next consecutive study, in 1994, added seven more to this group. Using the expanded parameter of 12 to 24 months versus 24 to 36 months, the cumulative data was 14 out of 15, which was substantially beyond the .001 level of significance.

The depressed patients in this study were severely afflicted, which may account for the surprising high penetrance of the symptom of hearing voices prior to 24 months. The data is startling, and demonstrates a high correlation between emotional trauma prior to the development of language centers and the subsequent language dysfunction of hearing voices. This applies not only to persons suffering with major depression, but applies to persons suffering with schizophrenia as well. The research has demonstrated a strong correlation between schizophrenia and emotional trauma prior to 24 months. When the schizophrenic returns to the mind and brain that was developing prior to the development of language, the left posterior superior temporal gyrus atrophies proportionately more than any other region of the brain, and the person has the language dysfunction of hearing voices. We believe the atrophy is a disuse atrophy caused by a shift to areas of the brain that were in use prior to the massive development of the language centers.

ADOPTIVE STUDIES:

In 1985, Davidson reported that 35 percent of the 160 emotionally disturbed adolescents at Elan One in Maine were adopted [as compared to two percent in the overall population]. This is statistically significant substantially beyond the .001 level. Most of these children, according to Davidson (personal communication) were adopted in the first two weeks of life. This points to a very early origin for this particular patient population, which excluded schizophrenia and was comprised of a mixture of conduct, identity, personality, impulse and substance abuse disorders.

Objections to the Elan One data center around the fact that wealthier families adopt more and can better afford a costly institution. A national survey by Childtrends (Zill, 1985) shows that 1½ times as many adopteds come from families with incomes of at least $25,000 (1981). Multiplying the number of institutionalized adopteds by two-thirds should compensate for this, but even if this were multiplied by a factor of one-third, the significance is still beyond the .001 level.

In the same year, 25 percent of the borderline children at the Institute for Living in Hartford were reported to be adopted. Angelones (1990) reported that the Institute's Borderline Survey of several area hospitals, including the Institute for Living, West Chester and Chestnut Lodge, revealed 25% adopteds among their borderline population. This, too, points toward a very early origin for borderline patients, and perhaps even during the first months of life, as with the correlation between adopted and the non-psychotic but emotionally disturbed patient population found at Elan One. Using data from Childtrends' broad based survey of 15,416 children, 15.1 percent of the 358 adopteds between ages three and seventeen had seen a psychotherapist, as opposed to 3.7 percent of those reared by both natural parents. Once more, this is substantially beyond the .001 level. And 42 percent of the 12 to 17 year olds (N = 47) who were adopted after age 12 months had seen a psychotherapist as opposed to 5.1 percent of those reared by both biological parents. Again, even with 47 matched pairs, the significance is well beyond the .001 level. It is further noted that the adopteds were compared to similar persons reared by both biological parents in a broad based cross sectional population and not to a population of super normals. These last two sets of statistical analyses conclusively prove, within the guidelines of statistics, a highly significant increase in emotional disturbance among adopteds as compared to children reared by both natural parents. The data represents a broad based cross section of children, some of whom are adopted and some of whom are not. Furthermore, the data is "hard data." Either the children were adopted or they were not, and either they had seen therapists or they had not.

Adopted children, by definition, have separated from their biological parents. We hold early separations to be very traumatic. We attribute the increase in emotional disorders, at least in part if not entirely, to the early traumatic separations. This is consistent with our findings. The above data is highly significant and it is sufficient reason to study every kind of separation at every age for correlations with the later development of serious emotional disorders. *In the last set of data there was more than an eight-fold increase in emotional disorders among those who were adopted after age one, as compared to those reared by both biological parents.* Numerically this is an even greater increase than we found for schizophrenia among those with siblings born between 10 and 18 months. This points to the circumstances surrounding adoption as being similar in severity to the birth of a sibling—which is not surprising. More data eventually will provide a mathematical relative degree of importance for each early trauma.

12

Short and Long Research Questionnaires

A. The Search for Infant Trauma

B. The Identification of Symptoms & Diagnoses

C. The Search for Precipitating Trauma in the Adult

GUIDELINES FOR RESEARCH STUDIES

Many persons reading this material will recognize both the fertile ground and the urgent need for research in this area of investigation. We, therefore, present general guidelines of what to search for, in hopes of attaining useful data that can be cumulative from one study to the next. We welcome all carefully gathered independent data for our national registrar.

BRIEF FORM:

The brief questionnaire is meant primarily to gain an overview and to determine statistically if there is a correlation between early sibling births and the later development of serious emotional disorders. This form has served its purpose but is presented here for historical reasons and for those who may wish to conduct a quick and easy survey on their own patient populations.

BRIEF QUESTIONNAIRE:

Historical Information:

1. Date of birth of patient_____

2. Dates of birth of next two siblings whether living
   or deceased_____ and_____

3. Adopted?   Yes_____ No_____

4. Patient is a single birth_____, twin_____,
   triplet_____, Other_____

Psychiatric Disorder:

- Schizophrenia? Yes_____ No_____

- Bipolar Disorder? Yes_____ No_____

- Major Depression? Yes_____ No_____

- With psychotic features? Yes____ No____

- Have Heard Voices? Yes_____ No_____

- Dysthymia? Yes_____ No_____

These patients are to be compared to healthy or supernormal individuals to determine the number in each group with siblings at specific ages.

NOTE: Date of birth of next sibling *must* be obtained for *each* patient, otherwise the data will be skewed—because a higher percentage of schizophrenics are unaware of birth dates of siblings.

The 1994 version of this study is to compare, for each diagnostic category or symptom, the number of siblings between 12 to 24 months versus the number of siblings between 24 to 36 months. This eliminates the need for a control group. With a large enough sample the same survey can identify peak age of origin and age range of origin for each symptom/disorder.

CUMULATIVE EXTENDED SURVEY:

This survey will attempt to identify three things: 1) the complete spectrum of early infant trauma and the relative degree of importance of

each at each age; 2) a precise set of symptoms and diagnoses that correlate with trauma at each age; and 3) the identity and relative degree
of importance of each subsequent trauma that precipitates the return
to the first.

As we gather large amounts of data and begin examining it in an
organized way, comparing various combinations and exclusions,
new insights will surface. The standard questionnaire will be revised
repeatedly as the analysis of existing data further guides and directs
future studies.

A. THE SEARCH FOR INFANT TRAUMA:

At the present time, we list for inclusion in any overall study that
might contribute to cumulative findings, items which would seem
most pertinent. Some of the items will elicit hard data and others soft
data. The soft data items are included because on a large scale they
may reveal insights and items to study more thoroughly. The items
have one basic common denominator: physical or emotional separation from the mother or primary caregiver which can be experienced
as traumatic.

The following is a suggested list of items about which to inquire.
Each potentially traumatic event from infancy should be examined for specific date and specific age of occurrence, whether it
is documented and how, whether it is estimated and the plus or mi-
nus range of the estimate, whether it was anticipated or sudden
and unexpected, whether it continued as a repeated or as a prolonged trauma, and how often and for how long, and whether
there were noticeable signs of distress in the infant, and what
these were and how severe they were.

Date of birth of patient?
Single birth?____ Twin?____ Triplet?____ Other?____
Date of birth of next two siblings, whether living or
    deceased____ & ____
Adopted?
    Date of separation from biological mother?_____
    Date adopted?_____ Age?_____
        (Documented?_____ How?____ or Estimated?_____)
    What took place prior to adoption?
        Foster homes? Date_____ Age____
            (Documented?_____ Estimated?_____)
        Fondling homes? Date_____ Age____

Nurseries?   Date_____ Age_____
What happened after adoption?
    Moved to new homes/families?   Date_____ Age_____
    (Documented?_____ Estimated?_____)
    More siblings?   Date_____ Age_____
        (Documented?_____ Estimated?_____)
    Adopted mother went to work?
    Date?_____ Age?_____   (Documented?____ Estimated?____)

(Age *always* refers to patients and should be given preferably in number of days old, e.g., 12 27/30 months, 11 19/30 months, etc.)

Birth trauma?
    Long difficult birth? Describe:
    Forceps?___   General anesthesia?___   When?_____
    Premature?___   Months of gestation?_____
    Birth weight?_____   Incubator?_____   How long?_____
Mother was alcohol dependent?   Drug dependent?
    When did she become dependent ?_____
    What age was the infant?_____
Father was alcohol dependent?   Drug dependent?
    When?_____ What age was the infant?_____
Mother had major depression?   Dysthymia?
    When?_____ What age was the infant?_____
    (Documented?____ Estimated?____)
    Postpartum depression?_____ When?____
        What age was the infant?_____   For how long?_____
        (Documented?____ Estimated?____)
    Mother had a psychosis?   Schizophrenia?
        When?_____   What age was the infant?_____
        (Documented?____ Estimated?____) For how long?_____
    Father had major depression?   Dysthymia?
        When?_____   What age was the infant?_____
        (Documented?____ Estimated?____)
    Father had a psychosis?   Schizophrenia?
        When?_____   What age was the infant?_____
        (Documented?____ Estimated?____)
    Mother hospitalized?
        What dates?_____
        Age of infant?_____
        (Hard data, if possible, from hospital records)
        (Documented?____ Estimated?____)

Father hospitalized?
    What dates?_____ (Hard data, if possible, from hospital re-
    cords)
    Age of infant?_____
    (Documented?____ Estimated?____)
Patient hospitalized during infancy?
    What dates? _____ (Hard data, if possible, from hospital re-
    cords)
    What age was the infant?_____
    Associated with physical pain?_____
    Without physical pain?_____
Family member killed?
    Who?_____
    When?_____ What age was the infant?_____
    (Documented?____ Estimated?____)
    (Hard data from death certificate?)
    Mother died?_____
        Date?_____ Age of infant?_____
        (Documented?____ Estimated?____)
        Who took over?_____ When?_____
        For how long?_____
        Was death sudden and unexpected?_____
        Was there a prolonged illness first?___
        Beginning when?_____
        What age was the infant?_____
    Father died?
        Date?_____ Age of infant?_____
        (Documented?____ Estimated?____)
        Who took over?_____ When?_____
        For how long?_____
        Was death sudden and unexpected?_____
        Was there a prolonged illness first?___
        Beginning when?_____ What age?_____
    Brother or sister died?
        Date?_____ Age of patient?_____
        (Documented?____ Estimated?____)
        Was death sudden and unexpected?_____
        Was there a prolonged illness first?___
        Beginning when?_____
        What age was the patient?_____
Important person (caregiver) left home?____
    Died?____

"Nanny"?_____
    Date?_____
    Age of patient (infant)?_____
    (Documented?___ Estimated?___)
Grandparent?_____
    Date?_____ Age of patient?_____
    (Documented?___ Estimated?___)
Aunt/Uncle?_____
    Date?_____ Age of patient?_____
    (Documented?___ Estimated?___)
Sibling?_____
    Date?_____ Age of patient?_____
    (Documented?___ Estimated?___)
Other?_____ Who?_____
Date?_____ Age of patient?_____
(Documented?___ Estimated?___)
Mother went to work?_____
    When?_____ What age was the infant?_____
    (Documented?___ Estimated?___)
Patient started daycare?____
    When?_____ What age was the infant?_____
    (Documented?___ Estimated?___)
    Did the patient seem to be upset at the start of daycare? (Yes, no, do not remember?)
Patient taken to a babysitter?
    When?_____ What age?_____
    (Documented?___ Estimated?___)
    Was baby upset? (Yes___ No___ Do not remember___)
Babysitters only came to the house?
    When?_____ What age was the infant?_____
    (Documented?___ Estimated?___)
    Was baby upset? (Yes___ No___ Do not remember___)
Familiar person stayed with baby in the parents' house?
    When?_____ What age was the infant?_____
    (Documented?___ Estimated?___)
    Was baby upset? (Yes___ No___ Do not remember___)
Familiar person stayed with baby in another house?_____
    When?_____ What age was the infant?_____
    (Documented?___ Estimated?___)
Parents separated?
    When?_____ What age was the infant?_____
    Mother was extremely upset?

When?_____   What age was the infant?_____
Baby stayed with mother?_____
Baby stayed with father?_____
Baby was relocated to a new house after parents separated?_____
Family moved to a new house?
  When?_____ What age was the infant?_____
(Documented?___ Estimated?___)
(Hard data from purchase agreement, etc.)
Catastrophe happened in family:
  Father lost his job?
    When?
  Family lost home?
    When?
  Mother discovers father having an affair?
    When?
  Father goes to war?
    When? (Hard data, date from military records)
  Mother goes to Gulf War, etc.?
    When?
  Father goes to prison?
    When?
  Mother goes to prison?
    When?
  Mother has to care for sick relative
    (grandparent, another child, etc.)
    From_____ age to_____ age
Any other event causing mother or primary caregiver to feel up-
set, insecure, depressed, causing an emotional withdrawal?
Specify?
Age? Duration?—or causing the mother to be away and there-
by resulting in a physical separation? Specify? Age? Duration?
Is this hard data, i.e., documented?_____ How?_____ Esti-
mated?_____ ±?_____

National events also can serve as parameters, such as the 1929
stock market crash or the beginning of World War II, etc.

As much data as possible should be gathered, and with great care
and accuracy. Factor analysis of the data will reveal which factors
and which combinations and which exclusions at which ages yield
the highest levels of statistical significance for each disorder.

Any disease category or symptom can be studied for an increased
frequency of trauma at a particular age as compared to the frequency

of the trauma at the same age among healthy or supernormal individuals. This is the research format used in the 1985 study.

Any diagnostic category or symptom can also be studied according to the 1994 format, comparing the incidence of the disorder or symptom associated with trauma over one age range as compared to another age range in the same group of individuals. This eliminates the need for a normal control group.

B. SEARCH FOR SYMPTOMS & DIAGNOSES:

A second portion of the questionnaire is to be filled out by the therapist, and the diagnosis—for the purpose of the research study—may require concordance of two or more experts. A list of symptoms and a description of the reality the patient experiences is of greater importance than the actual diagnosis, because diagnostic categories can be arbitrary, they are not necessarily related to cause, and they may change from one year to the next. The diagnosis of schizo-affective disorder, for example, was described in the former *DSM-III Revised*, as being confusing and controversial and "has been used in many different ways since it was first introduced as a sub-type of schizophrenia." *DSM-IV* revises the criteria still further. The symptoms, therefore, are more important to study than the actual diagnoses. They relate directly to the reality, feelings and behavior at the time of the trauma. A century later, the diagnostic labels will differ, but the age specific reality, feelings and behavior will not change.

Parameters to be Studied and Described:

In the search for a suitable scale of symptoms, attention was drawn to the carefully constructed scale for the Assessment of Negative Symptoms (SANS) Andreason (1983) and the Scale of the Assessment of Positive Symptoms (SAPS) Andreason (1984).

These remarkable rating scales for negative and positive symptoms of schizophrenia are very useful in determining the *intensity* or the *completeness* of the movement into the early time/age/region of the brain, and thus are useful for measuring change in severity of the disorder. Regrettably these highly refined scientific instruments are not designed to differentiate between *ages of origin* of symptoms. We also are not interested in severity of symptoms at any particular time; instead our focus is on the experience/behavior/reality that existed at any time during the illness and particularly at the height of the illness. Thus, the SANS and the SAPS serve a different purpose and we can only borrow from their content in a limited way.

Schneiderian first rank and second rank symptoms as well as the *DSM-IV* and ICD 10 criteria can be used for symptom checklists only. Each symptom or reality/behavior/feeling must be explored for its peak age of origin and age range of origin, until we are able to date the age of origin of any symptoms/disorder, and we are able to know in advance that a trauma at a certain age carries with it an "X" percent risk of developing a specific disorder later in life. Eventually diagnoses might be based on age of origin, because treatment and medication appear more specific to age of origin than to diagnostic category.

Schizoid, schizotypal, and schizophreniform disorders will be studied along with the schizophrenias for age of origin, to determine similarities and differences pertaining to origin. The ages of origin may be similar and the disorders may represent a partial chronic expression of an earlier time leading to aberrant development. Again we have no attachment to any particular result, and we simply await the data to reveal the answers.

The parameters we study are the ones that tell us most clearly the age of origin of the illness. We like specific realities—particularly ones that any two researchers might agree on—such as the delusion that a pet is answering the phone or space aliens are controlling one's mind. Certain realities are plausible only at specific ages and we are trying to determine ages of origin in this survey.

The following examples provided are not intended to be a complete list; they merely exemplify the parameter to be examined and, in general, they are given in developmental sequence from earlier to later. The developmental sequences have not yet been established because of lack of data in controlled research studies, but cumulative observations have revealed a trend that is included here by way of example. Each symptom the patient has should be listed, and gradually its peak age of origin and age range will emerge. If a symptom is not present for a category, move to the next category. Record only what is prominent, or definite, even though subtle.

1. *Impulse Control*: We propose a scale of 0–10. Most importantly, the researcher is to provide specific examples of impulse control. For example, with a suicide attempt, was it instantaneous on impulse or was it carefully planned? While this parameter also reflects severity of illness, the earlier the age of origin the less impulse control there is.

2. *Physical Movements* (these are very important for identifying age specificity. Some movements identify a specific age and other movements describe an age range. It is important to describe anything unusual that is not simply a reaction to neuroleptics):

   Head banging and rocking (in utero?)

   Violent thrashing movements vs. waxy flexibility

   Arms and legs move in unison

   Food is pushed out of mouth when attempting to eat (prior to learning to eat solid food)

   Sitting and staring for hours

   Walking with elbows extended (toddler, for balance)

   Arms pronated, hanging in ape-like position

   Racing about in constant motion

   Waddle type gait

3. *Delusions*: From the bizarre to the almost plausible.

   "A machine is controlling me."

   "Aliens implanted a device that is controlling me."

   "People on television are talking about me."

   "People are talking about me."

4. *Voices* (content, quality, plausibility are important):

   - The patient's entire existence centers around a voice heard inside the head which is an all encompassing communication with a very important person. (1st months of life, prior to the exciting discovery with the rattle, that the sounds come from outside the head?)

   - "There is a clicking sound that is signal from aliens to do something every time I have certain thoughts."

   - "Voices are telling me to harm myself."

   - "I think I hear someone calling my name." (21–23 months?)

5. *Flexibility*: From rigid, inflexible and concrete thinking, to somewhat malleable thought.

6. *Affect:* Totally empty, numb—to flat to full animation.

7. *Beliefs* (specific beliefs are exceedingly important, and while beliefs will vary, there will be age specific common denominators):

    "I can't walk." (12 months)

    "Animals can talk." (14 months)

    "People are talking about me." (20 months)

    "I am a horrible person." (26 months), etc.

8. *Behavior:*

    - Extreme, urgent, compulsive behavior—but not totally bizarre. (1st month?)

      - Smear feces, eat bees

      - Sleep all day, up all night

      - Egosyntonic "wetting diaper" (soiling clothes) while eating lunch

      - Running nude through sprinkler in front yard

      - Throwing food on floor

      - (List *any* idiosyncratic behavior)

9. *Sensations:*

    Pain around face, head, neck and shoulders

    Warmth in mouth and lips, coolness across nostrils, unusual sensitivity to odors

10. *Feelings:*

    Empty feeling

    Flat

    Angry/paranoid

    Frightened and withdrawn

    Depressed with psychotic features (21–24 months)

    Depressed with extreme self-blame (26–27 months)

    Depressed without extreme self-blame (30 months)

11. *Speech*:

    Bone piercing voice (like the howl of the baby magnified by the vocal chords of the adult)

    Rapid flat speech presented in bursts "machine gun tongue" (12–13 months?)

    Baby talk, whining tone of voice

    Pressure of speech (22 months?)

12. *Hygiene*:

    Smear feces in hair

    Messy diaper (strong odor of feces in underclothing)

    Lipstick smeared beyond lips?

    No bathing

13. *Attire:* from the bizarre to the odd or peculiar

    Shoes on wrong feet, not tied

    Socks different color

    Clothes mismatched

    Nudity in public is ego-syntonic

14. *Medicating:*

- Patient is totally unaware of when needs medication. He may take medication religiously out of fear of loss of control, but has no idea when he needs more or less (e.g., some catatonics).

- Patient is aware but fights taking medication

- Patient is aware of when he needs more medication and takes it on his own

15. *Medications:*

- Medications that worked:

- Medications that did not work:

It is important to list the medications that worked and the medications that did not work. We will probably find that medications are specific to trauma of particular ages, because the developing infant progresses through the phylogenetically older structures of the brain. For example, Haldol is a good medication for paranoid symptoms of age 14 months origin, but when applied to paranoid symptoms of 19 or 20 months origin it can move the patient deeply into a depression and is more likely to result in tardive dyskinesia. This is a clinical impression that lacks sufficient data for confirmation at this time, but it occurs frequently enough to note. Age of origin studies perhaps also will tell us when to use tricyclics vs. SRIs vs. MAO Inhibitors. This survey should help identify which medications are most suitable for symptoms of each age.

16. *PET Scans*: areas of activity of the brain likely will be different for persons traumatized at different ages, and PET scan data, when available, will be useful. It is possible that PET scan data, when studied and identified in this way, can help determine choice of medication.

Diagnoses:

The diagnoses can be taken directly from *DSM IV* and can be listed as primary or secondary. In addition to the psychiatric diagnoses, medical diagnoses should be included too, such as asthma, ulcerative colitis, rheumatoid arthritis, peptic ulcers, hypertension, eczema and neuro-dermatitis. It would not be surprising to find peak ages of origin for many psychosomatic and psycho-physiological disorders. Already we have cumulative clinical evidence of a correlation between asthma and trauma at age 24 months, but we have not conducted a definitive study to confirm or negate this finding.

C. THE SEARCH FOR THE SUBSEQUENT, PRECIPITATING TRAUMA:

In addition to identifying original traumas, the research questionnaire can also identify the precipitating trauma that caused the *initial* return to infancy. We again emphasize the initial acute illness because after the infant mind/brain has been awakened by a significant stressor, it requires much less of a stressor to reawaken it. The stressor for the initial psychosis is a major separation, rejection, loss, failure in the present which *signifies* the original experienced threat of separation, and which is sufficiently intense and similar to awaken the first.

Data gathered from this study could provide a rational basis for a hierarchy of stressors as they pertain to persons with specific emotional/mental disorders, instead of stressors listed according to how they might affect the average individual. The obvious first trauma to search for is the break up of an important relationship. Sometimes this is clouded by failures that naturally follow a movement into the schizophrenic process. It is important to look beyond these failures to find the true precipitating factor.

A group as well as an individual can become the precipitating factor for the *first* acute illness. For example, a child who exhibits precursors of schizophrenia may be rejected at summer camp. If the entire group ostracizes him, this can precipitate an acute psychosis. Sometimes an employer trying to get rid of an employee, with negative write ups and criticisms, can precipitate a psychosis or major depression by presenting a long series of cruel accusations. Since this comes from a person of significance and importance, it can represent the initial experienced rejection during infancy and therefore precipitate an initial acute disorder.

Starting school, encountering a critical teacher, being ostracized by a peer group, entering puberty (and anticipating certain rejection for sexual interests), breaking up a dating relationship, enduring parental divorce, separating from a fiance, lover, friend, spouse—all can precipitate mental/emotional illness.

It is noted that in former *DSM III-R* the breakup of a dating relationship is considered only a *mild* stressor for children and adolescents on Axis IV. To the vulnerable teenager this may be the stressor that most frequently precipitates a psychosis. Separation or divorce was listed as a *moderate* stressor for adults, but it may be the most frequent precipitant of a psychosis in the adult. This is not a criticism of the *DSM III-R* because it is clearly specified in *DSM III-R* that the severity of the stressor is based on what the "average" person would experience.

DSM-IV Axis IV addresses psychosocial and environmental problems that significantly contribute to the development or the exacerbation of the current disorder. But the evaluation of the stressors is again based on what an average person would experience. This appears to be a contradiction. The stressors that most significantly contribute to the development or the exacerbation of the disorder are not the same stressors that would even affect the average individual. In schizophrenia, depression or substance dependence, a slight rejection, the "EE" factor, or having to live with original family often are far more important stressors for perpetuating the disorder. Our survey data could identify which stressors precipitated and which stressors perpetuated the illness for each particular disorder. Stressors that affect the average individual are also important, but they are not the stressors that most significantly exacerbate the disorder.

It is important to search for all precipitating factors and to identify the relative degree of importance for each. This allows for prevention of a first psychosis, because therapy can be started in the person who is predisposed whenever a precipitating factor is anticipated or as soon as it occurs. Subsequent acute illnesses do not need as dramatic a precipitating factor, and usually are induced by continued family contact. When total separation from original family has been maintained for many months or years, renewed family contact is readily seen to correlate with rehospitalization.

Items for a survey are in the process of revision. We invite coordination of efforts and will supply a current list of survey questions to any serious researcher interested in participating.

III

PREVENTION

13

Preventing the Original Trauma

To the extent that early trauma are identifiable, it is possible through educational means to prevent a large number of early trauma from ever occurring, and to modify or attenuate the ones that can not be avoided.

The research design, described in the preceding chapter, allows us to establish a peak age of risk for each emotional disorder or disease category related to early trauma. Based on 25 years of clinical observations, early trauma is expected to account for a large number of disease categories, and in particular the schizophrenias and the depressions. Because of the unique research design, the most likely peak age and age range of origin/vulnerability is identifiable for each disorder/symptom, as well as the relative degree of risk for each type of trauma.

Ultimately, large scale objective studies will reveal a precise mathematical peak age of origin for each symptom or disorder related to trauma. We already have demonstrated statistically significant correlations between early experienced threats of separation and the later development of serious disorders, and based on cumulative observations it is possible to post-dict clinically the approximate age of origin of each symptom/disorder. This appears to be accurate to within a few months and soon will be tested in a clinical research setting. We do not yet have statistical data to validate all the clinical findings, but to not include the only set of predictions that exist—

and which are based on 25 years of cumulative observations—
would be falling short of the mark.

INFANT TRAUMA REQUIRING PREVENTION OR ATTENUATION:

Early traumas largely have one primary common denominator: a relative degree of physical or emotional separation from the mother,
which frightens the baby and may trigger primordial fears of abandonment and death. The cry response is present throughout the mammalian species. Mammalian infants need the mother for survival, and
without the mother they would die. Absence of the mother elicits the
cry response. This is a distress signal, and when the mother hears it,
she quickly returns. Both the cry of the infant and the response of the
mother are well entrenched in the mammalian brain. (MacLean, 1973,
1985) This has been necessary for survival in mammals since the an-
cestors of the duck bill platypus, and natural selection assures its perpetuation. Without this means of bringing the mammalian mother
and infant together, infants would die and the species gradually
would become extinct. Thus the fear of separation is "built in," and it
is part of a primary survival mechanism. Separation, therefore, can be
so frightening and can produce so much stress that it literally can lead
to death. Anaclitic deaths among humans were noted by Spitz (1945),
A. Freud (1953, 1954, 1963) & A. Freud & Bowlby (1960), and this has
been recognized in other mammalian species (Harlow, 1965).

Since separation from the mother is closely linked with survival,
we must pay particular attention to anything that can cause the infant to fear separation, as we explore the range of infant trauma and
consider its prevention.

Birth of a sibling has been recognized as a severe trauma having
profound effects (Margaret Mahler, 1979), (McKenzie, 1981, 1984,
1986a, 1986b, 1992, 1995). The authors estimate this may represent as
much as one-third of severe infant trauma occurring after age nine
months. **The prevention of serious mental disorders through the
prevention of initial trauma must take into consideration either
the spacing of children, or special ways of attenuating the birth-of-
a-sibling trauma in children who are born in close sequence.**

If one chooses to space children close together, then great consideration must be given to the introduction of the new arrival. For a
best case scenario vs. a worst case scenario (based in part on cumulative case histories but without statistical study), picture the infant
who is totally dependent on the mother—who then suddenly finds

the mother gone—and who even may be sent to a babysitter's house because the father is at work and is not available to care for the needs of a one or two year old. The baby is very upset at the sudden disappearance of the mother, is frightened, confused, cries in distress, and is desperate for her return. Then the mother returns, holding and feeding a new baby. Suddenly all fears may culminate in a dreadful realization; the first child experiences that it has been displaced; its whole world, its entire existence has been lost; without the mother to care for its needs, there is no life. The deepest fears of abandonment and death, developed over 150 million years of patterning of the old and the new mammalian brains, can be triggered. Few people realize the extent of this fear. Its meaning becomes lost and confused with such words as "sibling rivalry," "jealousy"—and other such attributes that have little or nothing to do with the absolute horror and terror that is being experienced. To seal the book for the worst case scenario, some infants or toddlers then are sent off to the grandmother's house when the newborn arrives.

To contrast this worst case scenario with a better way to handle the same situation, let us picture a family where the older child—as much as possible (depending on age)—is told about the new arrival and about the older child's future role in the family. The first child remains at home, with a close family member, when the mother (and father) is at the hospital. When the mother returns, she is NOT holding and feeding a new baby. She rushes to the first child, tells him/her how much she missed him or her, makes a great display of attention/affection over the first child, and then later introduces the subject: "Would you like to see your new baby brother or sister?" After the introduction, the mother again makes a big fuss over the first child and gives it gifts. Thus, by actions—that speak louder than words—the first is assured of its continued value and place in the family, and the threat of displacement and abandonment is substantially lessened.

This better case scenario was learned by the first author through an experience with puppies. We had an adorable Pomeranian puppy for three weeks and then decided it needed a companion. When the second arrived, the first snarled and pulled back. Instinctively I snatched up the first puppy, hugged it, made a big fuss over it, and when I set it down it wagged its tail and walked up to lick the face of the second. All it had needed was assurance of its own position before it could welcome the addition of the second puppy.

The worst case scenario was gleaned from histories of a number of patients who had schizophrenia or depression. The ideal is more hypothetical, based on practical experience and conjecture. While this does not represent scientific research, we must begin somewhere. If the trauma relates to the infant fearing separation, it makes sense to do whatever possible to increase the infant's sense of security, its sense of belonging and of feeling wanted.

ANTECEDENT TRAUMA:

As with posttraumatic stress disorder from adult life, antecedent trauma sets the stage for a more severe response to subsequent trauma. Sigmund Freud (1926) noted that preexisting anxieties or neuroses make traumatic experiences more acute. Burgess & Holstrom (1979), Hendin et al. (1983), Helzer (1987), and Hough et al. (1989) all note the same. Logic might dictate this as well. Anxiety and suspense cause the event to be more frightening. If one is among friends, in daylight, and someone attempts to startle him, consider the response—versus, if he is walking down a lonely path, on a dark night, full of anticipation and fear, and the same person attempts to startle him.

Thus, we must look to antecedent trauma that could cause the early infant trauma to be experienced as more severe. It is possible that all the second trimester assaults may operate in this way, including viral infections, famine, malnutrition, paternal death, toxins, and anything that threatens survival of the infant or upsets the mother. For references see *Second Trimester Factors* in Chapter One. Another major antecedent trauma is the birth trauma. A number of researchers have found a higher incidence of schizophrenia among those who have experienced birth trauma, for example, A. Grof (1985), Mednick et al. (1987), Dykes & Mednick et al. (1992), Cannon & Mednick et al. (1993). Trauma at birth has to be frightening to the newborn. Anoxia, brain injury, prolonged compression through the birth canal, near death experience—all must leave a mark. The average one year old still flashes back to the birth experience, which is why it fusses and screams when a tee-shirt is pulled over its head. An infant who is severely compromised with a near death experience at birth is even more primed for a later trauma to be more frightening.

In one family, the ninth of ten children had severe anoxia and brain damage at birth. All children were closely spaced and this one was 15 months older than the next.None of the others developed emotional difficulties, but when this one experienced a major separation later in life, there was a return to age 15 months reality. Had the person not experienced the brain injury at birth, it is possible that the age 15 month trauma might not have been sufficiently terrifying to allow for the reawakening as schizophrenia, 30 years later.

Birth trauma is not intentional and for the most part it can not be avoided. **Child birth education and good prenatal care can eliminate some of the trauma, but when birth trauma occurs, it should serve as a warning to make greater effort to avoid subsequent trauma,** particularly over the next 34 months.

A PREVENTABLE TRAUMA OCCURRING AT BIRTH:

The immediate clamping of the umbilical cord is one birth trauma/injury that has become common practice and which can be avoided. The immediate clamping of the cord prior to the infant taking its first breath has been shown to result in petechial hemorrhages throughout the brain in higher primates sacrificed at birth—as compared to ones in which the cord was not clamped (Pearce, 1977). After the struggle through the birth canal, the infant needs all the oxygen he can get and the pulsating cord is still an important supplier of this oxygen. Thus, it should be left intact until the lungs have been inflated fully and are working properly. Conceivably this anoxia and brain hemorrhage at birth could set the stage for later trauma to be more frightening. Both the birth trauma and the brain anoxia/hemorrhagic trauma are associated with a separation (birth), and this may contribute to setting the stage for later separations being more frightening. Just as childbirth classes and good prenatal care are important for reducing birth trauma, **prior discussion and planning are important for eliminating this unnecessary cause of traumatic brain hemorrhage.**

CIRCUMCISION:

Another trauma, occurring shortly after birth, is circumcision. This generally is done without anesthesia—because the baby is thought to be too young and therefore unable to feel anything. More accurately, it cannot say or do anything. Undoubtedly it is traumatic and likely it has an effect. If this trauma were to increase the incidence of schizophrenia appreciably, then there would be a much higher occurrence of schizophrenia in men than in women—which reportedly there is not. Nonetheless, this could be studied by evaluating male schizophrenics vs. super normal males and comparing the number of non-circumcised persons in each group.

Other disorders that are more common in males should be studied

for correlation with circumcision. This is particularly true with infantile autism. Currently great emphasis is placed on the neurological findings in autism, with the assumption that correlation proves
causation. This assumption is false. Some of the neurological change
may be the result of the disease process, just as it is in schizophrenia.

Autism is associated with conditions that have neurological le-
sions, such as congenital rubella, phenylketonuria, tuberous sclero-
sis, fragile X syndrome and Rett's syndrome (Kaplan & Sadock), and
it is associated with infant trauma in the first 18 months of life (Bettelheim). Most autistics are mentally retarded, language is poorly developed, about one-forth develop grand mal seizures and as many
show ventricular enlargement. Thus, a great variety of assaults to the
brain appear capable of producing the group of symptoms called autism. Severe early emotional trauma—possibly including circumcision—must not be excluded as a major factor. **Fixation and
continued activation of early trauma sites—to the partial exclusion of later developing sites, such as the language centers—also
can account for the symptoms of autism as well as the differences
in brain volume and electrical activity.**

There is growing evidence offered by the Pre and Perinatal
Association of North America that circumcision may represent a serious trauma to many infants. For this reason it should be studied using our methods. While the trauma of circumcision might or might
not heighten appreciably the later trauma of separation (depending
on how closely it is linked with separation), it could heighten subsequent castration fears during the Oedipal stage of development. Sigmund Freud described castration anxiety as existing in men and not
in women because women cannot be castrated. This explanation is
plausible and likely is the primary reason why males have castration
anxiety and females do not. Another possibility, however, is that
women do not experience circumcision, and circumcision could account for added fear of further cutting injury to the same part later in
life. A simple research study of circumcised vs. uncircumcised individuals, using an anxiety rating scale, could determine if this early
trauma indeed had an effect on the later development of castration
anxiety. **Until all correlations between circumcision and emotional disorders are studied further, we recommend against circumcision without anesthesia, and against circumcision or any other
painful procedure without the mother being present.**

OTHER EARLY TRAUMAS REQUIRING SPECIAL ATTENTION:

Preemies:

Premature babies are left alone in the hospital. While we do not yet have good data on the separation in the first weeks of life, those who were adopted in the first two weeks of life experience an early separation, and they also have a very high incidence of the later development of mental disorders, including borderline syndromes.

If it is possible to stay with the premature baby during its hospitalization, without sacrificing an older infant or toddler, this is the safest alternative based on present findings and projections. The emotional difference may relate primarily to the early separation from the mother. An interesting study would be to determine the number of non-adopted borderline individuals who were incubator babies and compare this with the number of non-adopted super normals who were incubator babies. If the origin of the borderline syndrome is in the first month of life, the study would confirm this. Until the completion of such a study, we recommend the mother stay with the baby until it is ready to come home.

Fetal Alcohol Syndrome:

This carries with it physical attributes related to the in-utero blood alcohol level. While a host of emotional/mental symptoms also are attributed to the in-utero blood alcohol level, more likely these relate predominantly to the lack of mothering or the inconsistency in mothering that occurs in the first months or years of life, as a result of the mother's alcohol dependence. For prevention, this may be a time for institutionalization of the mother while she is pregnant, and a time for a continued serious treatment of the alcohol dependence after the baby is born. Ideally, the alcohol dependent woman should be informed about the devastating impact of alcoholism on the baby, and she should have her alcohol dependence treated *before* she becomes pregnant.

Adoption:

Adoption should take place at birth, not two weeks later. Nine months should be sufficient time to make the necessary arrangements.

With adoption there already has been a major separation. Every effort has to be made in the direction of providing security, to avoid reawakening and inflaming the original trauma. Adoption must be reserved for the person who wants to be a full time mother to the baby. She must delight over everything the baby does—each developmental landmark, every new utterance, all "cute" behavior. The adopted baby has already endured one separation and must have the devoted attention of one constant mother figure who will be as close at hand as a mother bear with her cub. The busy professional who is not able to take time for a pregnancy and who plans to utilize a "nanny" or a daycare service to rear the child, should rethink the decision in light of our findings. The idea of having an adorable loving child must begin with one full time mother who provides for the needs of the child during infancy. The needs of the mammalian baby for the mother have been established and are deeply entrenched. The adopted baby has already been traumatized or injured and therefore must feel fully protected by having its needs fully met. **The adopted baby needs a devoted, full time mother, preferably beginning** *at birth.*

OTHER EARLY TRAUMAS CONTINUED:
OTHER PHYSICAL SEPARATIONS:

Histories of approximately 300 schizophrenics, and at least as many depressed individuals and borderline patients, have revealed other early traumas that occurred at ages that were specific to the expected age of trauma—based on the symptoms the patient experienced. For example, one patient whose symptoms matched those of a person traumatized at 24 months, was found to have moved into a new house at age 24 months. By using the clinically based expected age of origin, various other early traumas were identified. On occasion it was confirmed that the expected age of origin matched the time the mother was sick and was hospitalized, for example.

Combination Traumas: Pain Plus Separation From
Family Plus Separation from Familiar Surroundings:

If the infant/toddler is sick and hospitalized, this can be a multiple trauma. First, the pain or the sickness intensifies the need for the mother. The fear that accompanies the pain makes the child more vulnerable to separation. Furthermore, the child is not only separated from the mother for part of the hospitalization, but the child is separated from its familiar surroundings as well. If this occurs when the baby has stranger anxiety, the trauma conceivable could be even greater.

One parent described the look on the face of his oldest son shortly after his son had surgery at age 18 months. He knew then that something was terribly wrong. When the man and his wife divorced 16 years later, his son returned to age 18 months and spent the next 12 years in institutions. The surgery was the finest available and the surgeon went on to become one of the most noted in the land. Nonetheless, the emotional trauma eventually destroyed the mind of the baby (the parents were not able to follow the recommendation that would have brought about a total or near total recovery). **Thus, as a preventive measure, when the infant/toddler is hospitalized, the mother must go to the hospital and remain there with him. This is especially true when painful procedures are involved.**

A Second Child:

If there is another child at home under the age of 35 months, the mother must try to offer as much security, reassurance and support as possible to this child as well. The other child can stay with her or visit in the hospital lobby when the hospitalized one is asleep, and/or have telephone contact upon request. If the older child is very young and at an age of origin of schizophrenia or schizoaffective disorders, it could stay in the same room with the mother and baby. While many hospitals are not aware or tolerant of this need, it is necessary to insist because of the potential harm when the infant/toddler is separated from its mother.

When the mother has to be at the hospital and when it is impossible for the infant/toddler to be there with her, this is not a time for the father to place the infant/toddler in a daycare center or in someone else's home. This would be a double separation—a separation from the mother and a separation from home (which also represents a degree of security). A family member with whom the infant/toddler is familiar or attached, or preferably the father, should stay with the child in the child's own home. Ideally, the child should know that the caregiver will not leave until the mother returns.

In summary, physical separations are very traumatic to a child under two years eleven months, and the younger the child the more severe it can be. Thus, **physical separations have to be avoided or attenuated as much as possible.** This includes separation from mother and separation from home and separation from father. If the child is comfortable with the father, he may go places with the father as long as he does not exhibit signs of distress or withdrawal. One must not equate the vacant stare with not being upset. While this is not likely to occur when the infant is with the father, it certainly is present in the early daycare situation:

The Nine Vacant Stares:

One especially warm and intuitive woman psychotherapist, who reared four children of her own, described a particularly tragic modern day scene. She adored young babies and always made eye contact with them, in church and in other public places, and she was accustomed to having them respond with smiles, gestures and gurgling sounds. Out of curiosity she visited a modern infant daycare center for the infants of employees of a national bank chain. It was touted as the finest in the land, and the bank was regarded as being progressive, providing ideal care for babies of their working mothers. Nonetheless, this professional woman was horrified by what she encountered. There were nine babies, sitting around a table, staring blankly ahead. Repeatedly she tried to make eye contact with them, but to no avail. Each one simply stared blankly ahead. Nine vacant stares. The children had "adjusted"; they no longer screamed and fussed. One must wonder how many thousands of times this same scene is duplicated across the nation every day and what the outcome will be.

Since Chouchesku was executed in Rumania, a number of the 100,000 abandoned babies have been shown repeatedly on national television with a plea for food and blankets. The children were shown starving and literally withering away—but many of them were really dying of hospitalism or anaclitic depression. There were more than a few vacant stares. The looks on the faces of the abandoned babies werea terrible sight.

Babies **need the mothers**. Not just a diaper change and a bottle. The baby wants the mother to change the diaper and to hold the bottle. If there is no mother, then at least there has to be one constant mother figure. This was brought out by Anna Freud when anaclitic deaths in the foundling home were eliminated by assigning one nurse to ten babies—instead of rotating the caregivers. Whereas this prevented death, it can not be seen as ideal. Neither can daycare centers for babies.

Diminished Mothering:

When the warmth and nurturing is absent in one's own early life, it is difficult to pass it onto the next generation. Harlow (1965) showed that primates reared by terrycloth mothers could not relate well enough to one another to mate, and one that finally did simply batted away her baby when it came to feed. Dr. O. Spurgeon English (personal communication) pointed out that a woman who has had great difficulty in her early relationships with her mother, does not want to repeat the mother-infant experience with a child of her own, and usually avoids having children. Dr. John Rosen (personal communication) noted that geese reared without the mother did not know how to rear their own goslings. This led him to see the development of schizophrenia as an aberration in mothering. We are not that hard on mothers. We view the origin as an unfortunate set of circumstances at a crucial stage of development which results in the infant being traumatized by a fear of separation, abandonment and death. There are, of course, some women who did not receive adequate mothering themselves and who therefore can not provide it for their offspring. This prolonged difficiency in mothering is then passed on to the next generation. But if the mother is severely schizoid because of a lack of mothering, she is far less likely to marry and/or to have children. Thus, we do not concur with Dr. Rosen's concept of the "aberration of the mothering instinct" as being the primary causative factor in the development of schizophrenia. It certainly can cause schizophrenia, but usually the cause instead is a traumatic separation experience.

To prevent the lack of mothering, the mother must be available to the baby. Ideally, she should be happy, content, secure, and should delight in every developmental landmark and everything the baby does. When this occurs—i.e., when the baby has the opposite of the terrycloth surrogate mother—the chance of it developing full warmth and relatedness is maximized.

The prolonged stress of diminished mothering has to be contrasted with a sudden loss or separation from the mother, and has to be contrasted with the advent of intermittent mothering—as with daycare. The safest approach to child rearing is to focus on the needs of the baby for the first three years and defer the needs of the parent until later.

Intermittent Mothering:

Presently, most mothers are intermittent in that more than half of mothers with one year old babies are working and have placed their babies in daycare centers (Stains, 1987). In a survey of women psychiatrists (Wood & Paley, 1989), 50% returned to work before the babies were 3 months old, and 84% returned to work by the time the child was 6 to 9 months old. **The degree of trauma partly depends on**

whether the infants remain in their own home as opposed to outside their home, are with close relatives vs. with strangers, and
whether the substitute caregiver remains constant or is exchanged
or rotated with other caregivers.

Emotional Separations:

In addition to the trauma of physical separation from the mother and
diminished or intermittent mothering, there can be an emotional separation from the mother as well:

If the mother suddenly loses a close relative or the family loses
their house or the father loses his job or if the mother learns that her
husband is having an affair with her best friend, the mother suddenly can become very upset and emotionally leave the baby. If she suddenly has to focus all her attention on another child who becomes
sick, this can be distressing as well. **The emotional separation from
the baby can be just as impactful as a physical separation**, and at
times is even more perplexing to the baby. **Thus, if the mother becomes acutely distressed or distracted over any life circumstance,
she must make greater effort to turn her attention to the needs of
her baby.** This effort in itself often will have curative properties for
the mother. When energy is directed toward helping another, one's
own pain, needs and suffering are diminished (McKenzie, 1983).

SUMMARY OF EARLY TRAUMA:

Thus far we are looking at several categories of early separation from
the mother:

1. A sudden trauma that results in the baby's terror of separation
   from the mother, e.g., birth of a sibling, death of a parent, mother
   is hospitalized, or goes to war (e.g., mothers who had to leave
   their babies to go to the Gulf War).

2. A trauma to the mother that results in the mother's sudden emotional withdrawal (e.g., she may have another child who dies).

3. The terrifying event being heightened because of antecedent
   traumas—such as gestational trauma or a birth trauma.

4. The traumatic separation from mother being heightened because
   of concurrent trauma such as pain, separation from home, separation from all familiar people, and stranger anxiety.

5. Trauma of intermittent mothering—i.e., trauma of being reared by a daycare center five days per week. This may combine the initial terror of separation from the mother with the prolonged stress of not having needs met or not having needs met by the mother. Not having the mother present also may impact on development. Spitz (1945) reported that the mother is the one person best able to stimulate the infant. The natural response of the mother to delight over everything the baby does, is probably crucial for development. Dr. Suzuki taught the world that it is possible for a mother to teach a two or three year old to be an accomplished violinist by simply praising each small accomplishment. This is something that men, in general, are not as inclined to do or are not as capable of doing. If there is a baby in a room full of people, mostly the women come alive and fuss over the baby. They engage babies with gestures and sounds that may be a unique and important part of the mothering instinct.

6. Deficiencies because the mother experienced deficiencies in her own infancy, is schizoid, etc.—i.e., physically she is there but emotionally she is not entirely there.

7. Prolonged stress because the mother is alcohol or drug dependent, or is depressed.

Fathers:

Fathers can play an important role with the infant/toddler and often they do. In some instances the father can be more attentive, warm and nurturing than the mother and provide for the needs of the infant in a superior way. But on average, do they have the same mothering instincts? The same patience? The same attentiveness? Undoubtedly there will be some who do. Instincts are built in, however, and for approximately 150 million years mammalian babies have been reared by their mothers. Thus, it would be natural for the baby to prefer the mother and to prefer to have the mother meet its needs. The father should do all he can to help meet the physical and the emotional needs of the infant, but he can also help the mother feel happy and secure so she will be better able to do what mothers probably can do best.

Remedies:

Plan ahead.

1. Avoid the obvious traumas of separation as identified above. If

there is a problem with drug or alcohol dependence, or with depression, get treatment before having children.

2. Achieve sufficient financial stability in advance of having a baby so that daycare is not necessary prior to age three.

3. Anticipate the traumas that can not be avoided and plan strategies to lessen their impact as much as possible. With unexpected crises, always focus first on the effect on the infant and modify behavior accordingly.

Divorce:

Traumas associated with divorce rank high among infant traumas, because divorce is a multiple trauma. Usually the child is separated from the father physically and is separated from the mother emotionally—because she is upset and depressed. Sometimes there is also a separation from the home and from older siblings—all for the convenience of others. If parents were forced to study the effects of parental discord on their children, and if they were to recognize fully what happens as a result of separation and divorce—depending on the age of the children—they would set aside their own needs more readily and focus instead on the needs of the young. Considering the penalty they pay later in life, with children in and out of mental hospitals—or taking drugs—it is in the best interest of even their most selfish needs to attend first to the needs of the children.

When divorce occurs, problems are minimized if each parent focuses exclusively on the needs and interests of the child. When the needs of the children are made the primary concern, parents fight less and problems are reduced, but the impact on the infant/toddler/child/adolescent can be devastating nonetheless.

Child Abuse Agencies:

Child abuse agencies require checks and boundaries themselves. They can replace a bruise with a trauma that scars a young child for life. A child can be terrified when taken out of a home and away from his family. A family can be traumatized and intimidated by an agency out of control. Therefore, these public agencies must be closely monitored to see they focus on the needs of the child. Commercial groups can have divided interests. Businesses are run for profit. Agencies are susceptible to purposes of secondary gain, and have been known to be harmful to both child and family.

Combinations of Trauma and Prolonged Stress:

In summary, early trauma can be categorized in several ways: there are single moments of extreme terror, emblazoned in the mind at fixed points in time, and specific sites in the brain, subsequent to which the individual suddenly can return. There are multiple early traumas—some acting as antecedents, some serving to awaken and inflame earlier trauma, and some as multiple primary trauma sites—e.g., one for schizophrenia and one for depression—or, one for hypomania and one for a frightened schizoid withdrawal. Multiple traumas usually coalesce around one or two early sites, just as multiple war trauma coalesce around a few primary sites. With war trauma, this is evidenced by the fact that it is unnecessary to desensitize the individual to each trauma in order to desensitize to all trauma (Shapiro, 1989). After being desensitized to the first several, the person may be desensitized to all. In other words, *subsequent trauma and previous trauma coalesce around a few important major trauma sites. This appears to hold true with multiple trauma from infancy.*

Thus, there are single trauma at various ages, there are multiple trauma at multiple ages, there are single trauma with multiple components—such as physical pain plus separation from the mother, and multiple trauma with multiple components, and then there are prolonged stresses, such as having a mother who is severely depressed, or being left with a babysitter or a nanny throughout each day. Not only is there a prolonged stress of inadequate mothering, but there can be a developmental delay or deficiency because the baby needs the attention given—and which is best provided by the mother. The joy of the child is to have the mother delight over each new accomplishment. This leads to accelerated growth and development. The babysitter or the day care attendant might not be able to achieve as much, which can result in diminished growth and development.

The prolonged stress can be multiple, such as having an alcohol dependent mother who also works. It can span any period of time and be of varying degrees throughout the infant and toddler stages of development. This prolonged stress—when awakened later in life—can provide the basis for seeking oral fulfillment, such as with drug or alcohol dependence, in which the person continuously seeks to put something in the mouth to feel good.

The prolonged stress can be combined with momentary trauma when a sibling is born or when the parent goes to the hospital. Spitz (1945) showed that in some instances the children who already suffered a lack of mothering were not as affected by separations during infancy and they had a decreased incidence of anaclitic deaths. They may have been protected partially by not being as fully attached, but this does not mean they were healthier. No one fully knows the impact of a lack of good mothering, but this certainly is an area for further study. Based on cumulative clinical experience, we would correlate this with a lack of emotional attachment and warmth, developmental deficits, and a lack of basic trust (Erikson).

Not only can the prolonged stress fix a time zone to which to return, but it can bring about characterological differences that carry forward along the diagonal, developmental line as well—i.e., long before the person becomes alcohol dependent or has a dual diagnosis, he can develop dependency needs and other character defects that carry forward (See diagonal line in Appendix, diagram "D": Alcohol & Drug Dependence). Sometimes he becomes a "taker" instead of a "giver." But this can work in reverse. One schizophrenic, traumatized at age 17 months, watched his mother suffer a terrible depression when he was 2.2 to 2.4 years old. His enormous desire to help her and to ease her suffering at that age carried forward and caused him to try to help all suffering creatures, from the creatures of the forest to the handicapped on the streets of Philadelphia. The intensity reached saintly proportions, yet when he shifted to the 17 month brain/reality, there was extreme detachment and apparent cruelty, "apparent" because the adult portion of his mind/brain largely remained unaware of the enormous suffering of his victims (see Gary Heidnik, Section I).

Thus we have single or multiple terrifying trauma that serve as fixed points to which to return. We have prolonged stresses of various types and intensities for varying periods of time at varying ages, with or without single or multiple trauma of varying intensity and varying ages—all of which fix a moment or period of time, and all of which may carry forward along the diagonal developmental line and/or build at an unconscious level to be reawakened at a later age. Like PTSD of later origin, infant trauma can manifest as acute, chronic or delayed, or a combination of all.

NEW DIAGNOSTIC CATEGORIES:

Considering the multiplicity of the trauma, the multiplicity of the age, the multiplicity of the duration, the multiplicity of the combinations of traumas, ages, durations, etc.—it is little wonder that there are many diagnostic categories and that they overlap. Eventually, when the developmental nature of mental illness is more widely recognized, there will be a categorization of developmental disorders according to age of trauma. Clinical symptoms cluster around specific ages of origin and are useful for predicting severity of illness and prognosis. This type of categorization will also be helpful for prevention because it will heighten awareness that a certain set of symptoms relate to an experienced threat of separation from the mother which peaks at a specific month during infancy. This heightened awareness should spread and cause professionals and lay persons alike to be more attentive to providing for the needs of infants and avoiding feelings of insecurity and abandonment among them.

PREVENTION OF ORIGINAL TRAUMA THROUGH EDUCATION & PUBLIC NOTICE:

Prevention of early trauma has to take into consideration all possible early trauma, and the education of the public must be as extensive for emotional trauma as it is for physical trauma. Child rearing is an important project and takes careful planning prior to the birth of the child. The vast number of children who develop schizophrenia, depression, and drug and alcohol dependence as a result of early trauma should underscore the great need for such a program of prevention. Therefore any foreseeable trauma should be weighed and avoided as much as possible. The acute, intermittent and prolonged trauma and stress should be anticipated and avoided. When the inevitable sudden and unexpected trauma occurs, every effort should be made to attenuate the traumatic experience and desensitize the child/infant immediately. A lost parent should be replaced with a permanent substitute as soon as possible, for example.

Prevention must take place through education. More research is necessary to determine with greater precision the nature of early trauma and the ages of maximal vulnerability, but prevention must not wait until those determinations have been made. The preliminary findings, based on 25 years of cumulative observations correlated with case histories, indicate severe repercussions from certain early trauma and these trauma should be eliminated to whatever extent possible. The results appear to be potentially so devastating that one should not await further studies before taking appropriate precautions. The public, the parents, the educators and the mental health workers need to know now what the dangers are, and how to avoid them.

Health care agencies must be made aware, as well as adoption agencies, parents, the divorce courts and the hospitals. The general public needs to know, and this should be taught in schools and through public service announcements. Changes are necessary in regard to the common practices of the working mother and daycare. It is probably more beneficial to the economy of the family and the economy of the country alike for the mothers to stay home with their babies, at least for the first three years, and to separate gradually and only as the baby is able to tolerate the separation. This first level of prevention, the prevention of the infant trauma, is the most important level of prevention of all. It can eliminate or modify the early points or ages of fixation and thereby eliminate serious mental illness related to infant trauma. By avoiding the prolonged stresses of infancy and early childhood, the problems of alcohol and drug dependence can be reduced to the extent they relate to early prolonged stress. Even the elevated MMPI schizophrenia and depression scales and the alcohol and drug dependence that are associated with extreme war trauma and a return to the helplessness of infancy, theoretically could be reduced by eliminating trauma and prolonged stress during infancy.

──14──

Preventing a First Psychosis or Major Depression

We have seen a multiplicity of determinants—which vary in time, duration, age, intensity, number—and which result from such a variety of things as the mother catching the father in an affair, to the barn burning down. Yet all have the one common denominator: a relative degree of physical or emotional separation from the mother as experienced by the infant. This can be an actual physical loss, such as occurs in death; a fear of having been replaced, such as occurs with the birth of a sibling; an emotional separation, such as when the mother suddenly experiences a tremendous loss and begins grieving; or it can be the prolonged stress of a relative degree of physical and/or emotional separation, such as may occur with a schizoid, depressed, or drug or alcohol dependent mother, or even with a working mother.

IDENTIFICATION OF THE VULNERABLE INDIVIDUAL:

In preventing an initial psychosis, the first task is the identification of the vulnerable individual. The vulnerable individual is identified two ways: 1) by the history of infant trauma; and 2) by the appearance of the precursors of schizophrenia or other emotional disorders. Wide spread recognition of both is needed so that susceptible individuals can be identified and brought to treatment *before* a serious illness occurs.

Birth of a sibling or death of a parent during the crucial stages of development are the first and easiest trauma to recognize, and the age at the time of the trauma is already known and recorded. The parent has no guilt associated with the recognition of these particular early traumas and thus no resistance to identifying them.

The trauma of daycare or the working mother is harder to recognize because it stirs a sense of guilt, and for research purposes it is more difficult to date as well. Still other traumas are fleeting moments in time that soon are forgotten but leave their marks nonetheless. A mother can be devastated and depressed suddenly over an upsetting event or occurrence, and temporarily she may be absent emotionally to the baby. A year later the event may be repressed or forgotten—but the baby's fear reaction already may have been indelibly recorded.

Public education should start with the well-known early traumas and include a discussion of the wide spectrum of other events and situations that also can be traumatic. Equally as important at this second level of prevention is an awareness of the early precursors of schizophrenia so that potential problems are recognized before they become acute.

For example, a child who appears depressed or who has problems with separation—or who exhibits heightened needs—or who is devastated if a teacher is critical, likely was traumatized. The hyperactive child, the learning disabled, the loner, the bed wetter and the acting out child all may have underlying problems. Public education should direct attention first to the identification of the early traumas and then to the identification of the early warning signs.

In a study by Jones et al. (1994), schizophrenic patients were slower to reach motor milestones, and by age two more failed a developmental check. At age 4-6 more preferred solitary play, and checks by teachers at ages 10, 13, and 15, indicated they were more timid, avoided rough games and competition, and they daydreamed and appeared washed out and unhappy. These and other precursors need to be identified for all to recognize.

Teachers, clergy, preschool nursery personnel, pediatricians, psychotherapists—all need to become aware of early traumas and early warning signs of serious emotional/mental disorders, because something **can** be done about traumas after they have occurred and before the person has a first psychosis or major depression. The person who has suffered a terrible infant trauma **does not** have to develop a serious problem. The worst often can be avoided. Even after a severe early trauma, a first psychosis does not have to occur.

By conservative calculations, at least one in eighteen who has a sibling less than 24 months younger develops schizophrenia or schizoaffective disorder. This does not mean that only one in eighteen was traumatized by the birth of the sibling; it could be one in four or one in two. Since we do not know what percentage were severely traumatized by the birth of a sibling, we cannot determine what percentage of severely traumatized infants later develop schizophrenia. Longitudinal studies of infants whose mothers are about to give birth would be very valuable for determining the parameters of this particular trauma. This would also allow for the study of the development of schizophrenia from the early trauma to the precursors to the precipitating cause. At the other end of the spectrum from the initial trauma, is the subsequent trauma later in life that awakens the first. Not everyone traumatized at an early age has a *later* trauma that is sufficiently similar and intense to awaken the first trauma. *This is where level two of prevention can be most effective: When a subsequent trauma occurs, those who had early traumas or who exhibit the precursors of schizophrenia—and who have been identified and brought in for treatment—can be coached on what is happening to them, what to expect, and what to do so that a first psychosis does not occur.* Losing control of the mind is a terrifying experience. Being paralyzed by fear does not help prevent the complete progression into schizophrenia. Instead, it accelerates the movement into the terror of the earlier time. Fear is partly a fear of the unknown. Providing understanding eliminates the unknown and thereby eliminates some of the fear. It also helps the person plan, to avoid future rejections and failures, and to lessen the impact of subsequent trauma.

PREVENTION FOR CHILDREN WHO HAVE BEEN TRAUMATIZED:

With the very young who have been traumatized, great care initially must be given to provide security and protection, warmth, nurturing—so as to not awaken and inflame the original trauma. By the time the child is three to four years old, it can begin to understand a simple formula, told to the mother in the child's presence. This technique, of teaching the child, perhaps has not been described elsewhere—but it is very effective: If the therapist is talking to the mother about the child, the child will not miss anything—even if it seems to be distracted and is playing with toys. The therapist explains to the mother what had been terribly upsetting to the child as a baby, and why it would be upsetting to a baby. Then the therapist explains how an event in the present (e.g., a separation from the mother, to start school) awakens the first upset and causes a **partial** return to the feelings of the baby (along with symptoms such as bed-wetting, baby talk, and hyperactivity, for example). The child is provided support by the therapist when the therapist tells the mother that the child is not "bad," that this is just the way the mind works: an upsetting event in the present returns the child to an upsetting event in the distant past, and there is a partial return to being like a baby.

Next, the therapist provides goals that are ego-syntonic to the child (still speaking to the mother): "The child does not want to be a baby; he wants to be grown up." "He would not want to feel unhappy; he wants to be happy." "He does not want to worry about his mother leaving him; he wants to know for certain each time she leaves that she will return—and that maybe she will even have a little reward for him." Then suggestions are provided as to how to bring about these ego-syntonic goals:

The child will be encouraged to tolerate a ten minute absence, then a twenty minute absence. He will be encouraged to stop himself as soon as he can from a tantrum, because it only moves him deeper into the baby's rage—and he will be encouraged to identify and recognize thoughts, feelings and actions that belong to the earlier time. The approach of talking primarily to the mother is a very effective approach, at least through latency.

One four year old—whose mother was distraught when he was an infant over the discovery that her husband was having an affair—screamed mercilessly at her for attention. Constantly she had to repeat to him that she loved him, and constantly he insisted that she smile when she said it. He would sit in her lap, draw her lips in the shape of a smile with his hands and insist: "Say it nice." "Say it nice." That he was desperate for her approval was no secret, and the desperation matched the desperation of an earlier time, when the lack of maternal attention and approval was experienced as a threat to survival.

Therapy was difficult. When the mother began to interact with the therapist, the child would sit on her lap and insist she smile at him and talk nice to him and not be angry with him.

In between the screaming, the interpretations to her (him) were: "He wants you to be pleased, yet he does what upsets you the most...." "This is how upset he was as a baby when you were upset and could not give him the total attention a baby needs...." "To not get your full attention now returns him to when he could not get your full attention as a baby."

Gradually the interpretations shifted from cause to ego-syntonic goals to what he and she could do to achieve those goals. Over the course of three years, he made progress in terms of stopping the tantrum behavior on his own volition as soon as it started, and after four years of approximately 20 sessions per year, the child adjusted well in school and there are but few remaining signs of the return to infancy.

The mother is well trained in what to look for in the future. If her child experiences rejection or failure in school, he will likely need another interpretation—still to his mother—about how the present rejection returns him to the earlier experience of rejection as a baby (when his mother was upset). Further work with this child will not require as much time because it is primarily a matter of a review.

Again at puberty, with the arousal of sexuality related to hormonal changes—he suddenly can feel certain that he is bad and will be rejected. There also may be a flooding of emotion that may rekindle earlier emotionally charged experiences. The anticipated rejection at the onset of sexuality, combined with the flooding of emotion and a reworking of separation-individuation from infancy, accounts for a large percentage of schizophrenia and is how dementia praecox earned its name—as a dementia beginning at puberty.

After puberty, the next time he may require a review is when he begins dating. He will have to be forewarned about what feelings can be stirred when the relationships inevitably break up. It must be explained again at that time why he feels the way he does. He will have to be told that he will go through the painful separation process, perhaps ten times before he settles down with one person. For example, one recent tragedy could have been avoided very simply. An 18 year old boy (not in therapy) shot himself in the head because his girlfriend left him. It would have been a simple matter to explain how that separation returned him to age 2.3 when a sibling was born, and that to a two year old the mother is the whole world. If she leaves, it is the end of the world. To the adult, there are 5 billion people on the planet and if one chooses to leave, there is more than an ample supply of replacements. If he would have had this much understanding plus an awareness that he would go through a dozen more relationships before getting married, the tragedy could have been avoided.

Throughout adolescence, during each crises, there needs to be interpretations to prevent the first psychosis from occurring. If the child moves close to a psychosis, then even medication, along with a change in environment, can be utilized. The education process must continue and must include the shift in feelings/reality that could occur twenty years later if a marriage dissolves. Very aggressive treatment should take place if a psychosis begins, and this treatment would follow the guidelines for *prevention of a recurrence,* as described in the next section.

MORE EXAMPLES:

Another eight year old child was devastated because his teacher reprimanded him. In less than thirty minutes of therapy he understood perfectly well why he became upset, and he then explained his dynamics in terms of his mother (who suffered from schizo-affective schizophrenia, unipolar depressed type): "Oh, you mean it's just like when mommy gets upset, it's because something takes her back to being a baby when her sister was born." While the understanding undoubtedly allowed him to conceptualize the overall process and thereby reduce the upset feelings that he had, the mother was nonplused by his interpretation of her emotional problem, and she refused to bring him back. His future appeared brighter than hers.

In summary, when there is an early trauma, it must be identified by history or by recognition of symptoms, and then treatment must begin. The traumatized infant requires additional security and care at times of separation/stress. The toddler or young child needs explanations of how the mind works and interpretations of symptoms, along with ego-syntonic goals and helpful suggestions as to how to achieve the goals. Therapy is especially needed at times of stress, such as when starting school, going to camp, entering puberty and moving into important friendships and dating relationships that break up, changing residence and neighborhood, and, especially, such stress and trauma as parents divorcing. Many psychoses are precipitated when parents separate and divorce.

Vulnerable teenagers need to have important separations desensitized or attenuated in advance. They need to know that the present romance and probably many more will end and they will go on to still others. They need to be aware that only to the infant the world consists of ONE person. Awareness of the two realities helps keep the adolescent out of the "only one person in the world" one-year-old feeling/reality.

Parents who have a vulnerable child and who are thinking about divorce, should reconsider their own needs in light of the potential damage to the child. Countless vulnerable teenagers have become permanently institutionalized as a result of parental divorce precipitating psychoses.

Careful treatment, education and handling of the vulnerable individual can prevent a first psychosis or depression from ever occurring—which means the person might never develop schizophrenia or major depression. Education of persons who experienced prolonged infant stress can help prevent the development of alcohol and drug dependence—and intervention at times of maximal stress in these individuals may also have a preventive effect. The person needs to know that he can be prone to alcohol and drug dependence, and he needs to be forewarned about stresses that can return him to the infant-on-the-bottle mind/brain/reality. Education about the result of drug or alcohol dependence must be presented, clearly and emphatically— and substance dependence must be made ego-dystonic to the vulnerable child. Positive peer pressure and influence should be utilized in the adolescent age group. Any movement into alcohol or drug dependence must be interrupted, aggressively, and right away. With the first sign of substance dependence, the treatment must move into the prevention-of-a-relapse mode, and the problem must be treated aggressively as though the person has the disorder. The focus should be on getting the person out of the infant mind/brain/reality as fast as possible, as completely as possible and for as long as possible.

It is as though the other team has the ball at the goal line and it is about to make the winning touchdown. The therapist simply must stop the process before it begins. Substance dependence must not occur, and the moment it starts it must be interrupted—just as schizophrenia must be interrupted. The longer it persists, the more entrenched it becomes. Level three techniques of prevention must be called into play.

─── **15** ───

Prevention of a Recurrence

This is the third and final level of defense and the last defense for preventing a lifetime of mental illness. Until now, schizophrenia is rarely recognized before the first acute episode, and even then it is not diagnosed until six months later, because by strict definition the person does not yet have the disorder. Even when all symptoms are present, for the first six months it is called a schizophreniform disorder—probably because of the great reluctance to give someone the label of schizophrenia. In medicine the first sign of cancer is called "cancer until proven otherwise." Likewise, in the field of psychiatry, the first sign of schizophrenia should be regarded as "schizophrenia until proven overwise"—to emphasize the seriousness of the condition and the urgency for immediate, comprehensive evaluation and treatment. Let us set aside the diagnosis for all practical purposes, therefore, and start with the third level of prevention the moment the first **symptoms** of acute schizophrenia appear. That is what must be eradicated immediately and prevented from ever returning.

THE PRIMARY FACTOR IN PREVENTING A RECURRENCE:

In considering treatment for serious emotional disorders, ONE principle stands out above all. One principle holds more relevance than all treatment methods combined. One simple treatment recommendation, when strictly adhered to, can prevent a recurrence from taking place.

To understand this principle, we must return to the basic theoretical concept itself of the two minds in one skull. This principle is so

141

important that we have redefined schizophrenia as the co-existence
of two minds in one skull: the adult mind and the reawakened mind
(and brain) of the troubled infant. The definition itself tells something about the disorder that "split personality" or "split ego" does
not. It defines what the division of the mind is.

In applying this concept to treatment, let us consider the situation
of two persons in one room, one a child and the other an adult. If
there is a bowl of candy present, which of the two becomes excited?
Chocoholics aside, the child obviously is the one that gets into high
gear and clamors for the candy—because the child's needs are far
greater than the adult's.

The needs of the infant for the mother are immeasurably greater,
and these needs are heightened still further when there has been a
traumatic separation.

When the need-intensified infant mind is awakened and then
coexists with the adult mind, and the combination of the two minds
is in proximity of the mother, what has to happen?? Which mind
comes to the forefront and clamors for attention? The answer is obvious. Furthermore, the father and the siblings also are reminders of
the early life scene—and the infant had needs of them too. Thus, once
the infant mind has been activated by a trauma in the present similar
to the one in the past, any contact with a parent or sibling will quickly
reactivate the earlier mind/brain/reality. Even saying hello on the
telephone is sufficient to reactivate and perpetuate the disorder.

The recognition and understanding of the attraction and excitabil-
ity of the reawakened infant mind for the family member, along with
the absolute requirement of silencing the infant part of the mind,
makes obvious the Number ONE treatment principle: there must be
a complete and total separation and disassociation from all family
members in order for the infant mind to return to the inactive state.
Without total separation, the infant part of the mind struggles harder
to have its needs met, and the condition becomes more intractable.
This is highlighted with clinical examples in next Chapter.

The *re*activation of the earlier mind—once it has been activated—
follows a similar principle for schizophrenia, depression, delayed
posttraumatic stress disorder from adult life, and drug and alcohol
dependence. Very little is required to reactivate the earlier mind once
it has been activated.

When adult war-trauma is awakened, for example, even popcorn
popping will *re*awaken the earlier trauma and sound like machine
gun fire in the distance. The only difference is that the adult war-
trauma brain activity is located in the more advanced structures

instead of the phylogenetically earlier structures of the brain, as in schizophrenia.

In alcohol dependence, once the infant-on-the-bottle mind/brain/reality has been awakened, one drink will reawaken it. Similarly, with schizophrenia or depression, any family contact—subsequent to the activation of the process—*reactivates* the early mind. It is generally accepted that the alcohol dependent individual must separate from the bottle, but few recognize and accept that the severely disturbed must separate from the family. This is the Number ONE treatment principle and must be adhered to as strictly as the separation between the alcoholic and the bottle.

FACTORS AFFECTING SEVERITY AND OUTCOME:

The next three chapters explain in detail the deleterious effect of family on severity of illness and outcome. Other facts impact on prognosis and deserve mention. One that is not described elsewhere is age at the time of the original trauma. In general, the earlier the age of *origin*, the more severe and intractable the disorder. Psychosis from age 14 or 15 months is much more difficult to treat than psychosis from 20 or 21 months, for example. There is far more rigidity, delusional systems are more bizarre and intractable, and affect is noticeably more flattened.

Schizophrenia of earlier *onset* has a poorer prognosis too. It may begin in childhood or early adolescence *because* of a more severe propensity for the disorder, plus, those whose *onset* is early do not have a healthy normal period of adult function to which to return. Thus the therapist must make a particularly heroic effort to prevent the disorder from occurring in childhood or early adolescence, and this is especially true if the age of *origin* also is early.

Two more important factors are duration and remission. A prolonged uninterrupted disease process is far more intractable than an intermittent one with brief periods of illness alternating with higher levels of functioning. For this reason it is crucial to make every effort to get the person out of the infant mind/brain/reality as fast as possible, as completely as possible, and for as long as possible. A person who has been allowed to remain in a deep state of regression, for years, has a poor prognosis.

Psychotropic medications and daily activity programs prevent most persons from reaching the level of illness found in state mental hospital patients just 30 years ago. Without these interventions the hospitals might still be filled with severely regressed patients, and more would fit Kraepelin's description of the progressive nature and ultimate dementia associated with schizophrenia.

Treatment programs and neuroleptic medications still are only halfway measures, however. The two primary ingredients for prevention of a recurrence are: 1) a correct understanding of the mechanisms involved, and 2) a complete total separation and disassociation from original, nuclear family. In Section IV, which follows, this will be delineated carefully with clinical examples and supported by findings in the literature. New treatment concepts that evolved over the same 25 year period also are presented.

IV

TREATMENT

──16──

The Primary Principle, and Clinical Examples

Treatment considerations will focus on schizophrenia, but will also apply to depression, alcohol and drug dependence, anorexia nervosa, bulimia and all disorders stemming from the first 34 months of life. There is an interplay of treatment modalities from one disease category to the next, since the disease process is viewed as being similar. One principal difference stands out: for disorders related to very early trauma, especially prior to age two, the primary effort is to return the person immediately from the earlier mind/brain/reality instead of "abreacting" or "working through."

When the parallel nature of the disease process is understood, treatment modalities for one disorder can find useful applications in another. The hard won principles of Alcoholics Anonymous, for example, have wide application in the treatment of schizophrenia, and the primary treatment concept for schizophrenia greatly enhances recovery from alcohol and drug dependence.

THE PARENT-INFANT TRAP:

In Chapter XV, we made a bold statement that now calls for explanation, example and support from the literature. We held that separation from the original (nuclear) family was one of the two most important principles of treatment and the major principle for prevention of recurrence of serious emotional disorders. This view usually is not shared by family groups, mental health institutions or psychotherapists who have not studied carefully, in the same particular way that we have, the impact of family on the patient.

We present a method of study, along with observations from two and one-half decades of work, in order that the reader may study his patients in the way we studied ours and thus have an opportunity to evaluate our findings.

The recommendation of total separation between patient and family has nothing to do with blame for the emotional disorder, and we do not hold to the concept of the schizophrenogenic mother as the cause. The so-called schizophrenogenic parent is the **result** of the disease process; when the patient is traumatized and **returns** to the infant mind, all family members relate to him as though he were a baby. This is an automatic response and applies not just to the mother and the father and the siblings. To a degree it applies to all who come in contact with the patient. Mental health workers, psychotherapists and institutions are not excluded from this; they can fall into this trap just as readily as the family.

In some psychiatric institutions, for example, patients are allowed to stay up an hour later if they behave. Art therapists come to the units with crayons and coloring books, and in movement therapy, patients stand in a circle and pass around a big yellow ball. When highlighted in this way, it is easy to see the resemblance to a pre-school nursery. Patients are "taken" places and are spoken to like infants or very young children. While they are allowed candy and popcorn, they cannot have a beer. Adult functions are prohibited and rules are presented parent to infant.

One of the first principles of being an effective psycho-therapist in the treatment of serious emotional disorders is to never accept the parent role in a parent-infant relationship. Tenderness and caring does not require baby talk. While this can be a healthy part of intimate adult relationships, with the mental patient who is caught in an earlier mind/brain/reality, such an interaction will only serve to hold and keep him in his pathological state. If the therapist takes such a role, he may offer brilliant interpretations, but the patient will continue to experience infancy throughout each session.

To counter the automatic tendency to slip into a parent-infant relationship, it is helpful for the therapist to search for things a schizophrenic can do that the therapist can not. Often this is in the area of intuition—because schizophrenics can be very intuitive. If the therapist can recognize attributes of the schizophrenic which are beyond the ability of the therapist, this helps put the relationship on equal footing. Eventually it becomes second nature to relate to the schizophrenic only at an adult to adult level. To accomplish this, however, may require years of conscious effort.

Transitional programs are valuable, but most relate to the infant and try to teach the infant brain how to do things such as shop, cook, clean, wash, etc. It is better first to focus on getting the person out of the infant brain and then to encourage the adult brain do what it already is capable of doing. To relate at the parent-infant level and to try to teach the patient is to try to go in two directions at the same time.

Larry J:

Larry J., for example, was a 31 year old man who had just entered a transitional program and reported to his therapist that a nice nurse was going to take him shopping the next day to teach him how to shop. While this was much better than letting him sit in his apartment, it would have been more productive for her to have said "Let's go shopping together tomorrow and I'll see if I can give you some pointers." To say "I'm going to take you shopping tomorrow" places the patient in the child or infant role, inhibits learning, serves no useful purpose, and is not necessary. In the first two years he spent at the institution, he learned important coping skills but could have progressed farther if he had been treated as an adult. He was disciplined for the only adult-like thing he did—when he brought a six-pack of beer back to his apartment. He was told that he had to obey the rule of no sex—even though he was chronologically an adult and had his own apartment. While there are administrative obstacles to allowing otherwise, the no sex rule was presented with the emotional reaction one might have to sex in a preschool nursery. Relating to the patient as though he were an infant, and then trying to teach the patient how to adjust to adult life, is encouraging the patient to be an infant while telling him to be an adult. The patient came to treatment because he was in the two roles at the same time. Every therapeutic effort has to be in the same direction, to get him out of the infant role and into that of the adult. There is no place for baby talk and no place for preschool nursery activities in the treatment of schizophrenia.

MAINTAINING THE ADULT RELATIONSHIP:

The first author often prefers to treat schizophrenic patients away from the office, because the doctor patient relationship in a clinical setting more readily represents a parent-infant relationship to the schizophrenic. "Let's meet at the coffee shop" or "Let's go cut firewood,"—is a better approach. There is plenty of time for interpretation in almost any setting, and the therapist has more of an opportunity to observe the patient function in real life situations.

One schizophrenic girl ordered just a container of coleslaw for lunch and she never touched it. The next time she ordered a carton of milk and did not open it. How many therapists would be tempted to say "Eat your coleslaw" or "Drink your milk"? The correct response, of course, was to say nothing—not even "Are you trying to get me to say drink your milk? Do not accept the role. It is counterproductive. You do not want the schizophrenic to work through the problems of age one or two; you simply want to get the person out of age one or two. Seeing and relating to the person as an adult is helpful in that effort.

July 1991 the first author was asked to consult on a hospitalized schizophrenic patient. The patient seemed to comprehend the dynamics of his problem and was able to have a reasonably normal conversation. As soon as the patient's own therapist began to speak baby talk to him, however, there was a complete shift and he understood nothing. The patient's shift was immediate and dramatic. Address the baby and it will speak. Address the adult and the adult is more likely to respond. Thus, it is not just the parent who speaks to the reawakened infant. Often the institution and the therapist do as well—and this serves to perpetuate the disorder.

To summarize, we do not blame the parent for the cause of the schizophrenic process. On occasion, parents may be responsible, but far more frequently it is the result of an accidental, unrecognized trauma or an unfortunate set of circumstances at a crucial age of development. The so-called schizophrenogenic parent is a **result** of the schizophrenic process, and as to what the so-called schizophrenogenic parent does, the therapist and the hospital are doing too. In this sense, the term schizophrenogenic could be applied to the therapist, the hospital and the mental health worker—because all are responding to the patient as the infant, thereby enhancing the earlier role/relationship/mind/brain/reality.

Our effort to separate the patient from the parent has far deeper significance and reasons than any possible blame for the way the parent relates to the patient—because we would have to blame equally the hospital, the therapist and the mental health worker for those same reasons. **We separate the patient from the parent for the reason that AA separates the alcoholic from the bottle**—or for the reason the Vietnam Veteran separates himself from a busy, noisy, congested work place. We do not want anything to take the patient into the earlier mind/brain/reality.

CLINICAL EXAMPLES OF THE SHIFT TO INFANCY PRODUCED BY CONTACT WITH ORIGINAL FAMILY:

It is important to look at the clinical examples and to keep the patient in focus. Afterward we will examine documentation in the literature that provides supportive evidence for our findings:

Judy Z:

Judy was very helpful in the development of the concepts related to contact between patient and family. She presented a clear example in 1968, early in the practice, that was so dramatic that it set the stage for careful study of each family contact with each patient for more than the next two decades. Judy was hospitalized for extremely painful paranoid delusions. She "knew" everyone was talking about her and saying she was homosexual. She was terribly distraught and pained by this. Her suffering was enormous. The paranoid delusion lacked the bizarre quality of those derived from 13 to 15 months (i.e., there was no machine controlling her mind nor had a Martian implanted something in her brain). The delusion was the type found in paranoid schizophrenia of later origin—well into what we call the schizoaffective range—and it was accompanied by significant amounts of pain and depression. Her parents were not allowed to visit and the patient was kept on a locked ward where visitation was controlled.

She recovered quickly on the locked ward and was transferred to an open unit. After just one day suddenly she shifted to the full measure of her illness, crying, depressed and paranoid—and immediately she had to be returned to the locked ward. The parents had sneaked in to visit her on the open ward and the acute relapse followed spontaneously. Four more times she was transferred to the open ward and four more times the family came to visit which was followed by an acute relapse and a return to the locked unit. Finally the message was clear; everyone saw it and everyone began to cooperate. (Psychodynamically, when the parents came to the hospital she would shift to the infant. The infant was attracted to the mother—and therefore to other motherly figures—and this attraction to women was incongruous with the adult part of her mind. It was defended against by denial, and by projecting that others were talking about her and saying she was homosexual.)

At discharge from the hospital, this patient was recovered and did not return for treatment. From time to time persons who knew her reported that she was doing well. In 1991—23 years after the therapeutic intervention—she called to discuss another problem and reported that she had maintained the separation from the family, that she raised a family of her own, held a good job, had no recurrences of her very severe illness and never required medication following her one hospitalization. Without the separation, this would not have been possible; her symptoms were extreme enough that she would have moved more fully into the schizo-affective area of her brain and then deteriorated.

While it had been customary at many institutions to restrict visitors for the first several days or the first week, it was never the custom to restrict them permanently. The dramatic change in this patient each time the family visited, however, called for careful scrutiny of the process, and for longer periods of separation. For the next two decades, family encounters with every patient were carefully studied. In no instance, since the beginning of the study in 1968, did the contacts with family members prove beneficial. In each patient, each encounter—upon careful analysis—moved the patient further into the early process, deeper into the psychosis. Sometimes the change was dramatic and sometimes subtle; sometimes immediate and sometimes delayed. But the shift could always be detected:

Suzanne B.:

One schizo-affective woman had to be hospitalized when her husband left her. She functioned marginally after her recovery, and she reared her two children by herself. During some of her sessions she made a clicking sound with her tongue against her palate. She thought this was because her sinuses were dripping. But she was seen each Monday, Wednesday and Friday, and it only occurred on Mondays. Further questioning revealed that each Sunday she had dinner with her parents. On Mondays, there remained a sufficient shift to the infant-on-the-breast reality to cause the clicking sound heard in breast feeding, with tongue against palate.

Jack T.:

Jack had been diagnosed as having bipolar disorder, and had been hospitalized each year for ten years prior to meeting the first author during his last hospitalization. He had a classic bipolar I disorder, mixed type, and he had been on Lithium and Thorazine for ten years.

During this hospitalization, in addition to starting with medication and psychotherapy, he was encouraged to make a complete separation from his original family. As he recovered, all medications were tapered and discontinued. He began dressing the way he did in college and acting like a college student again. The changes were striking. After hospitalization he moved into his own apartment and found a job working at a courthouse. He bought a car, had a girlfriend, and worked successfully at his job for two years—all with no medication. On three occasions over the two year period, he exhibited a sudden partial shift to the hopeless depressed reality/feelings—which lasted only until the next interpretation. Each time it was interpreted that the shift could not have taken place without contact with his family, and each time he acknowledged a phone call to his family prior to the acute symptoms. Recognition of the dynamics immediately restored the sense of well being.

After two years of total freedom from bipolar illness and from medications, Jack decided to keep an insurance check that was intended for therapy and he did not return. This time when he contacted his mother he reestablished the relationship with her and rapidly deteriorated to his former level of dysfunction. For the subsequent 12 years he has been hospitalized almost annually, has been living in halfway houses and has been taking massive doses of medications. According to his present doctor, he has a chemical imbalance and must take his medication for the rest of his life. This undoubtedly is true. But when he maintained the separation he did not appear to have an imbalance and he functioned well without medication.

Sally J.:

Another patient had also been hospitalized each year for ten years prior to being hospitalized by the first author. She remained well with relapses only upon contact with her mother. Gradually, they stayed apart and she functioned well enough to live on her own.

After having no contact with her mother for approximately one year, a group of friends drove her to the Bar Mitzvah of a friend of the family. They reported she behaved appropriately and they were unable to detect signs of mental illness. Then her mother arrived late at the synagogue and sat down next to her. Within minutes, Sally began shouting obscenities and batting hallucinatory penises away from her vagina as she stormed out of the synagogue. She remained separated until just prior to her mother's death—at which time she visited her in the hospital. When her mother was dying and calling for her, she would say to her mother, "Sally was run over by a Mack truck"—and she would laugh. Apart from the inappropriateness she expressed then—and her idiosyncrasies that carried forward, there have been no recurrences, no hospitalizations, and no medications since the one hospitalization 15 years earlier. Contrast that with the ten hospitalizations over the previous ten years and the massive doses of medication that were required to keep her well.

Mary V.:

Mary was suffering from an acute paranoid psychosis and also had anorexia nervosa. She was a highly disturbed woman and required six weeks of intensive treatment in the hospital with large doses of medication and daily one hour psychotherapy sessions. After recovery, she returned to her husband and infant daughter. She adhered strictly to the recommended separation from her original family because her daughter was just six months old and she wanted to be able to rear her. Mary functioned well, and when her daughter was three years old, Mary went to work for a large pharmaceutical company where she held a responsible job for the next eight years. She even went through a nasty separation and divorce without further acute psychosis. But once each year for the first seven years, either she made a telephone call to her parents or they called her—and each time, within one to two weeks, she began hearing voices again and had to start taking medication once more.

Can you imagine what would have happened with family therapy? She certainly would have needed the family support system—because she would have regressed to infancy.

While in the hospital she looked at herself in the mirror and thought "My God, I'm huge." She was a tall anorexic weighing a mere 80 pounds. But to the mind of a 20 to 30 pound infant, the hulk of an 80 pound adult looked enormous. It was not necessary to treat the anorexia nervosa. When she was separated from her original, nuclear family, she quickly returned to adult reality and her weight returned to normal. Five years later she cured another anorexic at work in the same way. She said to a co-worker, "You seem to be having a problem"—to which the co-worker replied, "Mary, I'm dying." Mary suggested what had worked for her, and her co-worker agreed to a 30 day trial of separation from family. The anorexia disappeared—without further treatment.

In the same way, each patient shows some shift to an earlier mind/brain/reality upon contact with original, nuclear family members.

When trained to recognize this, a therapist will identify the subtle changes immediately.

Roseanne M.:

Roseanne had spent eight years in and out of mental hospitals. Not only did she have paranoid delusions in the schizo-affective range, but she had extreme depression, guilt and self-blame. Recovery was quick when the separation was adhered to during the hospitalization, but she could not keep from calling her mother, and after each phone call she cried in agony with guilt and self-hatred. Each time this progressed to paranoid delusions, requiring more medication. After the next hospitalization, she and her mother agreed to try the total abstinence concept, and she remained separated for one year. Her recovery was dramatic. Soon she was working and managed to buy her own car. None of the guilt and self-hatred was evident. She moved into a better apartment and began dating. There were none of the relapses into the infantile feelings and realities, and she required very little medication.

As Christmas approached it had been nearly one year of total separation and disassociation, and it was decided to allow a one hour visit. It was reasoned that if she became upset we could always return to the total separation once more. This was a fatal mistake. In retrospect it made as much sense as an alcoholic celebrating a year of sobriety with a bottle of champagne. It has been nine more years and Roseanne has never been able to separate again. She has gone through a series of therapists and has been hospitalized numerous times. It was a great therapeutic error to succumb to the seemingly reasonable request, in light of the holiday season, and to approve the visit. Once reawakened, the infant needs never could be quieted again. The driving force of the needs of the infant superseded any will on the part of the adult mind/brain to do what once had brought about a full recovery. The shift to the infant was too complete to ever lose its dominance again. Presently, she remains hopelessly lost in the abyss and torment of the infant mind, and she requires high doses of medication to function.

Many times the shift is not as dramatic. One attractive coed—who watched her diet conscientiously—could not understand why she ate ice cream by the half gallon each time she returned home for a weekend. Another patient missed work the Monday following a home visit on Saturday, and he previously had not missed work since recovering from his acute illness.

Henry T.:

Henry, after a dramatic recovery, gradually deteriorated when he moved back home to take over the family business. His trauma had been at age six months when an older sibling became ill and required all of his mother's attention. He was not delusional, but was replicating a classical state of anaclitic depression or hospitalism. He could mouth the words in monotone and clearly recognize "This is not me"—but could not recover from this state. He came out of his apartment only to drive to the office once each week. While he appeared to be making progress, he missed one appointment and then remained in his apartment. The family had to rescue him and take him to a hospital—where the second author took over and effected a recovery. With Henry, the movement into the psychosis after reuniting with his family was slow and insidious, and was not immediately apparent. Once he was deep into age six months, it was too late. The psychosis that resulted was severe and lasted one full year.

Larry J.:

Larry J., the first patient described in this chapter, also showed a series of very gradual disintegrations in his early treatment that never would have been attributed to contact with a family member had it not been for prolonged separation between contacts. Five times over the course of two and a half years he had a brief contact with an original family member, and each time he approached an acute psychosis four to six weeks later. Only late in his treatment was it learned that he felt an immediate "fuzziness" to his thinking. Each time this was followed a few weeks later by a looseness of association of ideas, and then words that rhymed took on the same or similar meaning, and ultimately after approximately six weeks this progressed to paranoid thoughts and ideas of self-reference. Had it not been for the fact that the same six week progression took place five times over the course of two and a half years, it never would have been recognized that each paranoid psychosis was preceded by a brief contact with a family member six weeks earlier. Once the sequence was recognized, it was possible to identify the initial feeling of "fuzziness," and start medications immediately after each subsequent contact. Such delayed responses as exemplified in this case have contributed to the poor recognition of the relationship between the contact with the family member and the shift to the infant mind/brain/reality.

After the sequence of contact leading to illness was recognized in

Larry J., he remained well and did not require hospitalization for seven more years. That hospitalization occurred when his mother decided to send him to a private community program that undoubtedly is one of the best in the country, with private apartments, visiting nurses, token economy, work training programs, daily group therapy, individual therapy, resocialization, and activities of daily living training. Tragically the program did not include the ONE principle, i.e., that of total separation, which stands out above all in the prevention of a recurrence. His mother was pleased to reestablish contact with her son once more, but he was rehospitalized four more times in the subsequent three years. No one even noticed or made a connection between the family contact and the worsening of his condition. It was too gradual and insidious for anyone to see. Instead of an occasional 100 mg. dose of Mellaril, he was medicated with high levels of Thorazine, Stelazine, Lithium, Zoloft, Tegretol, Valproate, Clozapine and more—all to no avail. In contrast, the first author cannot recall a single patient in the last 15 years—with the exception of severely regressed state hospital type patients—who required rehospitalization after gaining correct understanding and maintaining an absolute total and permanent separation from original nuclear family. In all 300 patients rehospitalization occurred only following contact with family members.

17

Factors Obscuring the Impact of Family on the Patient, and Support in the Literature

FACTORS OBSCURING THE IMPACT OF FAMILY CONTACT ON THE PATIENT:

Many factors cause the impact of family members on the patient to remain undetected or only partially recognized, resulting in a lack of awareness or appreciation of the magnitude of the effect on the patient.

A *delayed response*, such as in the case of Larry J., makes it more difficult to identify the correlation between family contact and a movement deeper into the illness. Usually the delayed reaction occurs within 72 hours, but in some instances the reaction is not detected for weeks. Even with short periods of delay, however, the correlation between the family contact and the mental illness routinely is missed. Not many, for example, would attribute failure to go to work on Monday to a family contact on Saturday.

Contacts may reawaken an immediate and dramatic return to the infant, such as with Suzanne B. in the synagogue—or the reaction might not be fully apparent until six weeks later, as with Larry J. Considering that most often contact with family is on a daily basis, while

159

the emotional reaction can last weeks or months, the therapist rarely has an opportunity to isolate the factor that produces the change. Thus, *the phenomena can only be studied and observed when there is prolonged separation from the family.* After weeks or months of no contact, the therapist must study carefully each change that takes place over the next 72 hours following even a brief telephone conversation. When studied in this manner, the changes will be apparent upon each contact, and the therapist will soon come to recognize even the subtle shifts into the infant reality. For example, there may be shifts in the level of hygiene, or the person—like the baby—may turn night and day around. There may be a phone call to the therapist in the middle of the night. This comes only from the infant mind and can be regarded as diagnostic. Never does the neurotic call the therapist at 3:00 A.M. This is limited to persons traumatized in the first 24 months of life. The baby does not hesitate to call the mother in the middle of the night, and this is one more of the subtle signs detected once the therapist begins to take note.

So far we see that the effect of the contact remains hidden because: 1) the contact is so frequent and the reactions last so long that the patient continuously remains affected by it. 2) There are delayed responses of up to six weeks before the full measure of illness is recognized. Thus no one sees the correlation between stimulus and response. 3) Frequently the changes are so subtle that they can be detected only after the therapist studies carefully the subtle changes that occur and learns to identify them.

Another major reason for failing to identify the reaction to contact with family relates to belief systems and to the therapist-patient relationship itself. Since the relationship with the therapist, the mental health worker and the institution is often a parent-infant one, the immediate reaction is to shelter, to protect and to nurture the patient as if he were an infant. To suggest a separation between the patient and the family is so contrary to the way one treats a baby that it simply is dismissed. The outcry is "But the patient needs the family support system." "Who else would take care of the patient?" "Who would shelter and protect the patient?" "Who would give him his medications?" "Who would see to it that he were properly dressed and groomed?" No thought is given to the possibility that if the patient were separated he might not have the disorder and maybe could take care of himself!

Thus, to suggest separating the patient from family is tantamount to suggesting a mother and her baby separate. This is the emotional response of the family, the patient, and the professional alike. Such unified reaction on all fronts is difficult to overcome. It is a natural emotional response that requires analyzing in the observer, otherwise the most important treatment dynamic might never be noticed.

Other reasons for non-recognition of the effect the family has on the patient relate to group pressures. Groups such as Families Unite for Mental Illness have become active and influential in the field of psychiatry. Because of the unfair criticism and the blame the parents have received over the years, this group is quite vocal about anything that does not attribute schizophrenia to an act of God—such as a chemical imbalance, a hereditary disorder, a virus or a brain disease. To suggest separation between patient and family sometimes is taken to imply that the parent is at fault and is doing something wrong—even though it does not imply that at all. In fact, the theory exonerates the parent altogether. But our primary recommendation of separation from family blocked earlier recognition of the concepts by family groups and those who would seek their acceptance and approval.

SUPPORT IN THE LITERATURE:

The work of G.W. Brown, referred to in Section I, lends strong support to our findings. Brown (1966) evaluated 339 post-mental hospital patients to determine what factors in the post-mental hospital environment caused the patient to return to the mental hospital. One factor alone stood out, and that was whether the patient returned home to live or went anywhere else. To be certain, the patients who returned home were with people who genuinely were concerned and cared, but, nonetheless, the ones who returned home were the ones who returned to the mental hospital.

From this research began the study of what it was in the family that caused the recurrence of the acute illness. Expressed Emotion, or the "EE Factor" soon was singled out. It became apparent that a low EE Factor was less harmful than a high EE Factor. This would be comparable to lighting a small firecracker next to a combat Veteran instead of a big one. But to simply try to reduce the EE (Expressed Emotion) Factor is—in another sense—like a person who has cancer and who wants to get rid of most of it. It would appear to be a halfway measure. Schizophrenia is a serious illness and every effort should be made to get rid of it completely, totally and right away. A *ZERO* EE Factor is immeasurably superior to a low EE Factor, and the ZERO EE Factor is brought about by a complete and total separation and disassociation from the original, nuclear family. In the first author's experience, approximately 75 of the 300 schizophrenic patients adhered to the recommendation of total separation, and of those patients, almost none had to return to the mental hospital. Furthermore, at least 3/4 of these patients required no more medication. This was not intended to be a scientific study, and consequently there is no tabulation of data to which to refer, but in looking back, practically none of the patients who maintained the separation had to be rehospitalized, and each patient who did require rehospitalization did so only after having contact with the original family. We now have affidavits from patients highlighted in the clinical vignettes and are in the process of reviewing hospital records to further validate our findings. This will be available on request.

EXCEPTIONS TO A GENERAL RULE:

The authors, over the 25 year period, have heard numerous objections to the general rule of separation, and have heard the same objections expressed many times. The most frequent objection is: "What about the state mental hospital patients? Aren't they separated from their families?"

Here we have to consider other factors: 1) recovery requires two components: separation plus correct understanding. Therefore, how much correct understanding did these patients have?; 2) how separate are the state mental hospital patients? Do they have visitors? Do they make occasional telephone calls; 3) how long have the patients been sick and how deeply were they allowed to regress? Ideally we prefer to bring the patient out of the earlier mind right away. If the illness were to persist and the regression were to become complete or nearly complete and the brain were atrophied for a prolonged period of time—or if the illness started in childhood, then, of course, there would be far less chance of recovery. But the persons who present for therapy before they reach an irretrievable state are different. They are still reachable and a recovery is likely. It is noteworthy that this population includes persons who, in former years, would become state mental hospital patients. Earlier treatment, widespread use of neuroleptics, and day programs have prevented a large percentage from the extreme regression seen in most state mental hospital patients.

MORE EVIDENCE IN THE LITERATURE SUPPORTIVE OF SEPARATION:

Much has been written about the biochemical changes in the older schizophrenic, partly as a means of explaining why not many schizophrenics come in for treatment after age 50. Here again the biochemical changes may be the *result* of the disease process and not the cause. Not many 50 year olds have parents, which we believe is why not many 50 year olds show up for treatment for schizophrenia. When the schizophrenic process is no longer active, it stands to reason that the chemistry changes as well.

CLINICAL EXAMPLES:

Clinically this is apparent. In 1988, the first author received a phone call from a 56 year old woman who said, "I had schizophrenia all my life and then it disappeared three years ago." His reply was "Yes, and you lost your last parent at that time." The woman confirmed that this was correct. The same year a proprietor of a restaurant, upon learning of the first author's profession, proceeded to tell about having schizophrenia for five years and then overcoming it. The author made the same post-diction commentary and once more this proved to be correct. After presenting a lecture in Madrid, April 1984, entitled "The Anatomy and Psychodynamics of Psychosis," the first author was approached by a woman in her fifties who said, "I never understood why, but when my parents passed on I had the feeling of an enormous weight being lifted off my shoulders." Thus, once more, both the literature and the clinical findings support an improvement in the disease processes when the parents are no longer present.

HOMELESS SCHIZOPHRENICS:

In a study by Katan (1990), it was found that homeless schizophrenics were more likely to return to being homeless if they were placed in the homes of original family members as opposed to other living arrangements. This work collaborates the findings of G.W. Brown and further highlights the impact of family on the schizophrenic.

INSTITUTIONAL COLLABORATION:

By chance, a hurricane destroyed one of the mental hospitals in the Virgin Islands, and the patients were sent elsewhere for treatment.

Placement was found for a large number of them in Pennsylvania. Much to the surprise of persons handling the program, even the patients who had very serious disorders and had been difficult management problems proved to be relatively free of symptoms when they were totally separate from family.

Another group in Israel is having similar success treating schizophrenic patients from the United States. These examples are fully in keeping with our expectations. For many patients, schizophrenia exists only in relation to family, and in no instance has family interaction proved more beneficial than complete separation and disassociation.

18

Separation as It Applies to Depression, Alcohol and Drug Dependence, Post-traumatic Stress Disorder, "Normals" and "Neurotics"

SEPARATION AS IT APPLIES TO DEPRESSED PERSONS:

Separation applies not only to the treatment of schizophrenia, but to the treatment of depressed persons as well. Suicidal teenagers respond in the first 24 to 72 hours and often show no signs of depression after the first two days—as long as they are provided with correct understanding and adhere to the total separation.

John D.:

John was a troubled 16 year old who contemplated slashing his wrists with a razor blade because of extreme depression. He was hospitalized immediately and the mechanism causing his suicidal depression was explained to him in approximately one hour. He understood the return to age 2-1/2 when his younger brother was born, and he understood how this was reawakened ten years earlier when his parents separated and he moved to California with his mother. He also understood how the constant contact with his mother after she and he returned to Philadelphia kept the earlier disturbed part of his mind active. Within 24 hours of hospitalization, there were no clinical traces of depression remaining. No medication had been used, and medication could not have worked as quickly. After approximately one week in the hospital, John suddenly was extremely depressed once more, reaching the same intensity of suicidal thoughts and feelings. Upon questioning, it was learned that he had received a telephone call from his mother earlier that day. This occurred twice more and each time it was immediately interpreted. Finally he recognized the pattern and realized that he could have no further contact with her.

For some reason, contact with his father did not produce the movement into depression, and John was able to live with his father. One day, when John had his foot bandaged after a slight accident, John saw his mother from across a parking lot and she pointed to his foot as though to ask what had happened. He had not seen her for nearly six months, and this is the only contact they had. Within hours he became suicidal once more and he had to be reminded that the contact produced the reaction. The suicidal feelings and deep depression lifted after approximately two days. At no time did John require any medication, and except for brief episodes following the contact with his mother, there were no signs of depression.

After enjoying recovery for approximately two years, John reestablished a relationship with his mother. Finally he was able to move in with her without becoming suicidal, but the close association caused him to give up his life goals of becoming a professional athlete and resulted in a depression that was not as severe. The depression was managed with Prozac for the next four years.

It is noted that in the treatment of depression of origin later than 24 months, it is possible to reunite the patient with family without a shift into the full extent of the disorder—as long as the patient is not also substance or alcohol dependent. Such reuniting has not proven beneficial, however, and living in the same household is definitely counterproductive.

Mueller et al. (1994) compared 176 persons with major depression and alcoholism to 412 with major depression alone, and found the latter group had twice the likelihood of recovery. His finding supports ours, in terms of difficulty in recovery from depression in dual diagnosis patients. In addition to having to recovery from two problems instead of one, the alcohol dependent individual may be reexperiencing stress from prior to 24 months, which would further explain the additional requirement of separation from family.

Another finding may be suggested by the previous example of the depressed adolescent who functioned and felt better without contact with his mother, and by adolescent patients in general who have a marked reduction in symptoms upon separation from original family. Tricyclic antidepressants have proven useful in the adult, and numerous studies have demonstrated statistically significant results. But as of 1993, the statistical significance has not been proven in children. After studying our findings, one factor becomes obvious; children live with parents—which keeps them locked into the earlier mind/brain/feeling/reality—and this works against recovery. Thus, according to our observations, tricyclics cannot be expected to achieve the same results in children as they do in adults, because children live with parents.

SEPARATION AS IT APPLIES TO ALCOHOL AND DRUG DEPENDENCE

Alcohol dependent individuals also are affected by family contacts. They must remain separated both from the parent and the parent substitute, the bottle. Fifty percent of persons dependent on alcohol have contact with one parent every day, and this serves to perpetuate their disorder.

Joseph P.:

Joseph is alcohol dependent and lives with his mother and his wife and three children. In 1990, Joseph took a vacation with his wife and children to Puerto Rico. There he managed to control his alcohol dependent condition. Upon returning home, he was back on the bottle once more. His mother went on a two week vacation and he stopped drinking altogether until she returned. When she returned, his infant needs were reawakened by her and he immediately started drinking again.

In 1986, the owner/director of several alcoholic treatment centers in the northeastern sector of the United States, was asked what happens when the recovered alcoholic returns home to live with original nuclear family. He chuckled and answered unhesitatingly: "He goes right back on the bottle."

No one questions the alcohol dependent's other separation—i.e., the separation from the bottle. But the separation from the parent may be one of the most important steps toward achieving this. The same holds true for drug dependence.

SEPARATION AS IT APPLIES TO POST-TRAUMATIC STRESS DISORDERS

To the extent that extreme war trauma awakens the total helplessness of infancy—causing an elevation of the MMPI scales for schizophrenia and depression and leading to an increase in drug and alcohol dependency—then separation should prove beneficial in the treatment of PTSD as well. Contact has the effect of increasing all of the infantile states and dependency needs. Every conscious effort must be made to get out of the earlier mind/brain, and this may include separation from family.

EFFECT OF SEPARATION ON THE "NORMAL" AND THE "NEUROTIC"

Children mature more quickly when they leave home—whether it is to go to college, travel abroad or join the military. Somehow they are better able to leave their childhood behind. Not only can the original family keep a reawakened infant mind active, as in schizophrenia, but continued contact with the original family serves to perpetuate childish needs, feelings and behaviors that were never fully extinguished in the normal individual. Young couples get along better with one another when they live separately from their families. Continued close contact may stir needs of early childhood, resulting in immature behavior not compatible with marriage. Periods of separation are helpful to the growth, development and maturation of the normal individual, but growth and development can take place without separation—albeit at a slower pace. Likewise, separation from original family enhances the progress and maturation that takes place in the course of psychotherapy with non-psychotic and non-substance dependent individuals, but therapy can take place without separation—although it is less efficient. Separation only becomes critical when the origin of the problem is early, especially prior to age two—as with the psychoses and substance dependence, when an earlier developmental part of the brain takes over.

WHICH FAMILY MEMBERS?:

Initially the focus was on the mother because the original relationship of the infant was with the mother. She was the all important one. Soon it became apparent that the father could elicit the same response.

Keith S.:

The importance of the father's role in the perpetuation of mental illness was first noted with Keith—a young acting out schizophrenic who was in and out of jail. The father was a retired physician who had a heart condition, and his life was devoted to worrying about Keith. Keith would call him at 3:00 A.M. from a phone booth in a dangerous neighborhood, and the father would rush out and retrieve him. At the hospital, he brought candy and cigarettes to Keith on a daily basis. The contact kept Keith sick. Each contact resulted in a worsening of his condition. Subsequent observations of other cases confirmed the fact that the father could have the same impact on the patient as the mother.

Siblings:

David B.:

David had been in the hospital 12 times and it was not clear what caused the recurrences of his schizo-affective range paranoia. He lived alone with his widowed sister who had reared two children and suffered from major depression herself. Finally his nephew—who moved back home with his mother—made it clear that he wanted David to leave. Ultimately David moved out on his own.

Over the course of the next three years there were no more psychotic episodes. Then David was hospitalized for a surgical procedure. After returning from the hospital, his sister moved in with him for a few days to help him "just to make him a sandwich and pour him a glass of milk." Within a week, he became acutely paranoid, was convinced he really had cancer and everyone was lying to him, and he left the country. Two months later a postcard arrived from Canada saying "checking things out up here," signed "David."

Relationships with siblings were scrutinized more carefully after this clinical experience, and it became apparent that they had an effect similar to that of a parent. It was speculated that older siblings might have a more pronounced effect than younger ones, but younger siblings have been observed to precipitate recurrent illnesses too.

Children:

One professional woman was hospitalized for schizo-affective schizophrenia, unipolar depressed type, with drug dependence. Each time she had contact with one of her children she became acutely disturbed. It was the same parent-infant relationship, but she took the infant role in relation to her grown children.

Aunts, Uncles, Grandparents and Others:

The safe approach is total separation from all. Schizophrenia is a serious illness and the top priority is eradicating it. If the therapist is attuned to subtle changes, there may be occasional brief contact with distant relatives to observe for changes—but if there are other alternatives, the contact is not worth the risk. One patient made a spontaneous recovery when he went to live with distant relatives in Spain, but he relapsed two years later when he returned home.

SUMMARY OF CHAPTERS 17 AND 18:

In summary we have offered theoretical reasons for separation, clinical examples illustrating the effects of contact vs. separation, and supportive articles in the literature showing better health and longer recovery if the contact is less or nil. We hope no one takes this as an indictment of the parent, for it is not. An alcohol dependent person is adversely affected by a bottle of scotch—even if it is the finest bottle of scotch in the world. The first glass takes him deeply into the infant world. Similarly, contact with any family member returns the schizophrenic to the mind and brain that was active at a particular traumatic time during infancy.

─────19─────

Treating the Patient

This section does not focus on what is known and is well described elsewhere. It highlights the application of the theoretical concepts to various treatment modalities, and it outlines new dimensions and approaches to treatment which may be of interest to the reader.

Separation and correct understanding are the cornerstones of successful treatment and recovery from serious emotional disorders. But there are additional factors and modalities, of course, including the judicious use of medications, the occasional administration of ECT, the cross referencing of adult and infant realities, the immediate identification of relapses each time there is a contact with a family member, the use of day programs, of work, school and community services, the therapeutic alliance and the personal interaction with the patient.

CROSS REFERENCING THE REALITIES:

The therapist must become an anchor in adult reality, a person with whom the patient can relate at such a firm adult to adult level that contact with the therapist immediately brings the patient back to the adult reality. One catatonic, in the excitement phase, was thrashing about uncontrollably as four police officers tried to restrain him. When the first author appeared, the patient continued to struggle in violent thrashing motions resembling the thrust of the infant in the birth process. While he could not stop the thrusting motion of the body, the rational part of the mind responded to the sight of his therapist and he explained in lucid fashion everything that happened to

171

him that day that led up to the loss of control. Just as his family represented his anchor in the infantile mind/brain, his therapist represented his anchor in the adult.

The identification and cross referencing of realities is a very important aspect of treating schizophrenia, and especially the paranoid. Wil Menninger (personal communication) once cautioned
"always start with the reality the patient is experiencing." This is
sound advice. One approach is to say "I absolutely believe, 100%,
that what you are telling me is exactly what you experience to be so."
"You are experiencing that people on television are talking about
you," etc.

Once this is fully acknowledged, it may be possible to move on to:
"The way we experience things varies somewhat from time to time
and from person to person. If ten people witness the same event, they
experience it ten different ways. If one person experiences something at ten different ages, he experiences it ten different ways. If you
are asleep and dreaming and a bear is chasing you, it is real until you
wake up. If you are hypnotized and told you are a rooster, that is real
until you are no longer under hypnotic suggestion. Likewise, when
persons shift to earlier ages, they may be experiencing what is real to
them at an earlier time.

"What you experienced to be real yesterday is not what you experience to be real today" (this interpretation is vitally important as the
patient's delusional system begins to change with the advent of hospitalization, separation from family and the administration of neuroleptic medication). "Perhaps what you experience tomorrow will
be different from what you experience to be real today."

As treatment progresses and the patient comes to recognize the
shifting realities, he can begin to recognize where the other realities
come from. One recovering schizophrenic woman complained that
when she returned from shopping she would put the groceries on
the floor instead of in the refrigerator. She did this even though she
knew the food would spoil. She, therefore, wondered why she did it.
It was easy to point out that the baby plays on the floor, puts everything on the floor and never puts anything away.

In a similar fashion, each symptom that is a replay of the reality/
behavior of the infant can be interpreted. When the patient lists
countless reasons why he cannot move away from his parents'
home, this is the infant mind speaking. The adult will find just as
many ways to make the separation possible. Every thought, word,
action, and feeling can be identified as to its source. Eventually the

patient learns to cross reference his thoughts and learns to recognize which part of his mind they are coming from.

What is real to the person depends on the reality the person is experiencing at the time. Only with special attention to cross referencing various realities can the patient begin to recognize "I've been here before." One of the best times to do the cross referencing is when the patient is coming out of the delusional system and the realities are changing on a daily basis. This is also a good time to identify how the particular reality or behavior relates to that of an earlier age during infancy.

One schizophrenic high school student whose mother just left home, partially returned to age 18 months when she left him at that time. His means of getting her to pick him up during infancy was to have a smelly diaper. His later symptoms were the same. He did not become overtly delusional, but his affect was flat and the stench from unclean underwear was so strong that no one could sit next to him. (Note: this first symptom was regarded by the first author as "schizophrenia until proven otherwise," and an aggressive treatment approach prevented development of the full disorder.)

Each symptom such as this needs correct interpretation until the patient has good understanding and comprehension of his illness. With schizophrenia of very early origin, interpretation can be more difficult since rigidity, concrete thinking and inflexibility are greater at earlier ages. More of the interpretations have to be made when the person is not in the acute state. To achieve positive results with the more disturbed, the total separation from family is absolutely essential otherwise there will not be sufficient return to the adult brain to allow for insight and recovery.

SHOCK TREATMENT:

Section One provides an example of the judicious use of shock treatment in the man who was afraid of hitting himself in the face with his fists—and then who later shifted to the anoxia at birth. While this patient had been given a lengthy trial of medication, this is not always the most conservative approach. There may be times when clinical judgment will dictate immediate shock treatment because it will bring the patient out of the psychosis sooner. If one can stop an acute psychosis the moment it starts, that may be the most conservative thing to do.

Another uncommon use of shock treatment is when the patient

has reached a plateau and does not seem to be progressing. With shock treatment the patient may brighten up and exhibit more affect. There may be a more complete return to a pre-psychotic level of functioning.

Contrary to the usual sentiment about psychotherapy while the patient is receiving shock therapy, the first author has found it useful to meet with the patient an hour per day during treatment to discuss the progress taking place, the goals, and to offer support and encouragement. When the patient participates in the attempt to reactivate the adult mind and brain, there is an atmosphere of mutual cooperation and a greater degree of trust. Empirically, this seems to bring a better result.

WHEN NOT TO GIVE SHOCK:

If the patient plans to continue contact with original family, there is little point to bringing him more fully out of his psychosis. The contact will assure recurrent illness and the patient will have to be medicated. It seems pointless to use extraordinary measures to bring a person out of a psychosis only to do what will cause a recurrence.

The literature points to recurrence of the schizophrenic condition after recovery with ECT. But research has not been conducted on persons who are shocked and then totally separated from original family. These persons would not have the same relapse rate. While our sample is small because of the infrequent use of ECT, those who recovered and remained separate from family did not relapse.

MEDICATION:

This, too, depends on separation from family. If there is no separation, a solid course of medication is essential. With a reduced expressed emotion (EE) factor, the need for medication is somewhat less. But with a *zero* EE factor, brought about by total separation and disassociation, and combined with correct understanding, usually there is very little need, if any, for medication. Within a few weeks, the same dose of medicine makes the patient drowsy and it must be reduced. After two months, approximately 70 to 80 percent—according to cumulative observations, not a research study—require either very little medicine or none at all. And they do not relapse as long as they maintain the separation. But one brief phone call to a family member can return the patient to an acute psychotic state. It is equivalent to a recovered alcoholic taking a drink. For a period of time he has no thoughts about taking a drink—and then suddenly the infant mind takes over and he cannot stop.

COMMUNITY SUPPORT:

Ancillary help is also important. The patient needs to keep active and to interact on all levels. He needs to be involved with as many groups as possible and with the healthiest groups possible. He may interact in halfway houses, yoga ashrams, chess clubs, softball teams, churches, synagogues, bowling leagues, health spas, ski clubs, etc. The progression is from hospitals to halfway houses to schools, jobs, social clubs and community organizations. Separation from original nuclear family helps each step of the way. Therapeutic community programs are well described elsewhere. We highlighted the importance of the adult to adult patient-therapist relationships in such groups and the need for non-regressive adult activity. The use of a well trained social worker to spend a few hours each day with the patient, visiting him in his home, introducing him to community programs and activities, looking for work situations with him, accompanying him to a job, and in short, reintroducing him to the world of the functioning adult—is an invaluable adjunct to the treatment of schizophrenia. Many patients simply need to get back on the right track after a prolonged illness. They need someone to go with them to the social security or the medical assistance office. They need someone to say "let's look at the newspapers to see what kind of jobs there are for you"—and then to go with them to the interviews and to the jobs until they are back on track. In this way the patient is introduced to the real world and not the make-believe. Instead of the "let's play store" approach utilized in some of the treatment programs, the patient is introduced to a real job and is helped daily to get there until it becomes routine. The patient also needs guidance and help in dating relationships and sexual relationships. These areas often are ignored but they are important aspects of adult life.

LOVE ENERGY:

Another dimension of help comes from clear identification of love vs. need. Movement in the direction of intensifying feelings of love is movement in the direction of reaching the adult mind. Movement in the direction of giving up needs is movement in the direction of giving up or letting go of the infant portion of the mind. Caution must be exercised in love relationships because for at least the first year after an acute psychosis the person needs stabilization before chancing another major loss, rejection or separation. This is a general rule taken from AA and applied to the treatment of schizophrenia. In AA, persons are encouraged to not form intimate relationships for at least the first year, since emotional entanglements can result in intensification of needs and then relapses.

For the same reason, it is important not to risk failure in school or in a work situation until there is recovery followed by a period of stabilization. Work can be very therapeutic, but the patient must not be set up for a failure. Strong guidance and support is required in matters of love, work and school.

It is exceedingly important to be able to identify love versus need in every thought, word, action, feeling. The patient who is disappointed or "crushed" by a relationship that is not progressing as he would choose, for example, must be helped to recognize that the upset feelings have *nothing* to do with caring about the other person; they have only to do with caring about the self and wanting the other person all for the self. The simple recognition of this truth allows the person to give up the attachment with much less pain.

Love is redefined to the patient as an attention or energy directed outward, and the byproduct of which is happiness. The opposite is need or desire, which is an attention or energy directed back to the self, and the byproduct of which is *un*happiness. Reverse the direction of flow of attention or energy and one has the opposite feeling. Fall in love and you are in a state of bliss. As soon as you want the other person to love you, you are miserable.

When the patient is miserable in a relationship, this is attributed to need and desire. The patient is encouraged to care and do for others, with no attachment to anything in return if he prefers to have happiness. The depressed person often is helped the most by careful delineation of love versus desire, happiness versus unhappiness. Age specific needs are also delineated. It is easier to dismiss needs when they are identified as relating to age one or two, for example.

RELIGION:

Most patients have some religious beliefs and many are very religious. The therapist who does not use religious concepts to help strengthen and reinforce treatment may be missing an extraordinary therapeutic opportunity. Once the patient has gained an understanding of the love energy concepts, if he has religious beliefs he can be encouraged to work diligently at intensifying his love for his creator. This is the safest of all love objects. He can fall in love and never risk rejection. The feelings of love can provide enormous energy, peace, bliss, happiness. These are ingredients that are not likely to be found in a pill. Sigmund Freud (1961) once wrote that the effectiveness of the therapy of the future may depend primarily on the mobilization of energy. Love is what mobilizes that energy. When a person falls in love he can work day and night, but when the direction of flow of energy is reversed, with the attitude of oh woe is me...aches and pains, etc.—the person can have so little energy that he can hardly move. While we cannot delve extensively into the love modality of treatment and the therapeutic use of religion in this volume, we must point out that this can be an important part of treatment and will be thoroughly discussed in a subsequent work.

SPIRIT WORLD:

If the patient believes in a spirit world and is hearing voices, make use of this. Be flexible. You may identify the voices as evil forces in the spirit world trying to influence, harass and destroy him. It is easier to get rid of voices and intrusive thoughts when they are identified as something external. And the spirit world concept is more manageable than the delusion that certain people are putting thoughts or voices into one's head. It is important that the patient dismisses the voices as soon as they occur. This is in keeping with the concept of getting out of the infant mind as fast as possible, as completely as possible and for as long as possible.

ADULT BRAIN ACTIVITIES:

Once free from family, the patient is encouraged to do adult things, such as play the piano, drive a car, read, use a computer/word processor, or even play computer games. This exercises the prefrontal cortex, which must become more active. The patient is encouraged to increase social skills by taking dancing lessons and joining social clubs. He is encouraged to keep a full schedule. He is encouraged to intentionally try to increase his level of responsibilities, such as doing his own laundry and grooming. This is made ego-syntonic. He is encouraged to increase his level of adult functioning and to avoid infant behavior, such as turning night and day around. He is encouraged to do everything to activate the adult brain and nothing to stir that of the infant. He is encouraged to force himself to keep on a schedule with deadlines. He is encouraged to gain a talent, a trade, to attend school as soon as he is able, and to exercise his mind and brain as much as possible. He is encouraged to work around his handicap. He is encouraged to recognize his limitations and to work on overcoming them and to focus on doing what he can do well.

EXPANDED RANGE OF CONSCIOUSNESS:

The patient is encouraged to learn techniques for functioning at a slower brain wave frequency and encouraged to learn to use the creative levels of consciousness for problem solving. In a study of 75 severely disturbed individuals, most of whom were schizophrenic and had been hospitalized, we conducted clinical evaluations as well as objective psychological testing before and after the 40 hour Silva Mind Control training course (McKenzie and Wright, 1981). We were looking to see who might be affected adversely by the training—which teaches people to go to a deeper level of consciousness and teaches how to use the mind at the slower brain wave frequency. We were surprised at the dramatic improvement in the patients when they learned to function mentally at a deeper level of relaxation. The objective test scores on the Experiential World Inventory, by Osgood and El-Meligi, showed striking change. Clinically there was much improvement and sometimes delusional systems cleared. While the training itself is not a therapy, it can be used as an important adjunct to treatment if the therapist is supportive and understanding of concepts and methodology.

THE BEGINNING OF TREATMENT:

Treatment begins with correct understanding which is presented in a matter of fact way during the first session. The patient is taught the mechanisms of the mind—as described in Section One. Not much history is taken. The patient is simply told what the illness is, what caused it, what the mechanisms are, how it works and what to do about it. This is presented in a very positive way: "It is not necessary to have this disorder. I will explain it and you will understand it." Usually the patient does understand within the first hour—which comes as a great relief after searching for many years and finding no understanding other than: "a chemical imbalance," "a brain disease," "hereditary," "a biopsychosocial disorder" or "many diseases with many causes."

During the session the patient usually is told the approximate month of origin of his symptoms, based clinically on the way he expresses himself and the reality he experiences during the hour. If the origin is the birth of a sibling, there is immediate confirmation of age of origin. The clinical estimate usually is correct to within one month more often than it is off by a month. This is convincing to the patient. Then his primary symptoms and reality are explored and these are related specifically to what the infant experiences to be real at the particular age at which he was traumatized. Gradually the concepts become easier for the patient to recognize.

A diagram of areas of activity of the brain is used to illustrate the differences between the normal brain with its increased prefrontal cortex activity versus the schizophrenic brain with its shift to earlier developmental areas of activity (See Appendix, Diagram "F"). Early in treatment—from the very first session—we make it an ego-syntonic goal to get *out* of the infant brain and back into the prefrontal cortex of the adult. The patient is told that the cerebral atrophy will reverse because it is a disuse atrophy. It may relate to a softening or a partial demyelinization of brain tissue [prior to destruction of cells]—but will reverse with exercise. Clinical evidence for this is the fact that the cognitive impairment in the schizophrenic reverses with successful treatment. Supportive evidence is found in the brain studies that indicate the brain atrophy associated with alcoholism reverses after six months of sobriety (Carlen et al., 1986). All this is presented in a very positive light. The therapeutic alliance begins during the first session. Family members are encouraged to attend the first session—unless a complete separation already has been accomplished. Everyone needs to understand because everyone must cooperate with the total separation from family.

The patient and family are encouraged to first try 30 days of separation—and if that works, extend it. It is almost guaranteed that there will be breaches in the agreement of separation. A parent will just happen to be driving by or will have no choice but to drop something off or to call for a very legitimate reason. The patient will go home to pick something up and to get his mail, or he will return home because he is out of money, etc.

Each time this happens there will be a setback. The observant therapist will be able to tell right away and point out to the patient "You are a little more upset today. Was there some kind of contact with the family?" Each time there is contact there is a retreat into the infant mind/brain/reality/symptoms, and each time this must be pointed out. Gradually the patient begins to recognize the repetitive shift into the infant brain, and he notes it himself when it occurs. At first he does not make the connection because of the delayed response. He may talk to a family member on Sunday—and then on Monday he experiences that people in school are talking about him, and he is angry at them and blames *them* for his being upset. This sequence usually occurs and is pointed out several times before the patient and family begin to recognize and appreciate more fully the impact that family contact has on the patient. Identifying symptoms of regression related to family contact, pointing them out and winning the complete cooperation of patient and family is the greatest therapeutic challenge. Once this is achieved, usually there is no further need for medication.

V

MENTAL HEALTH REFORM

—20—

Laws Governing Treatment

Mental health reform must be based on sound understanding and must maintain an awareness of the two minds that coexist: the warped, twisted, distorted, irrational mind of the troubled infant, and the clear, logical, rational mind of the adult.

Presently, the law listens to the mind that speaks, and when the angry, bizarre, irrational one year old mind takes over, that is what dictates the treatment for both. In other words, there is no protection for the healthy adult mind when the infant mind is in charge.

Patients may predetermine whether or not they will receive extraordinary medical treatment if they become terminally ill and are unable to speak for themselves, but they cannot predetermine psychiatric treatment in event they lose control of their minds and have no ability to think or reason. Because of present law, they are forced to rely on the irrational one year old mind and brain to make their medical/psychiatric decisions. Patients at least should be able to predetermine that the doctors will use whatever extraordinary measures are necessary to bring them out of psychoses.

Preferably, the laws should take a firm step back to earlier times when doctors were allowed to treat the patients by whatever means necessary. Such regulation still applies in general medicine: if the heart stops beating, apply house current to the chest—or rip the chest open and perform cardiac massage. But if the mind stops working, ask it what type of treatment it wishes to have. This is less sensible than the illogical thinking of the deranged patient.

Regina J.:

In 1974, Regina J. became acutely psychotic for the first time. She was hospitalized immediately and against her will. When she refused to take Thorazine orally, the first author said "okay, every time you do not take the oral dose of medication we will give it to you by injection." Soon Regina agreed to take the medication orally.

Next, she signed a 72 hour notice and said she was leaving. She was told "okay, you are allowing only 72 hours to get you well, so that means shock treatment is necessary. You are scheduled for shock treatment at 8:00 A.M." She rescinded her notice and overcame her acute illness within an additional ten days. Her adult mind was thankful afterward. The infant was virtually annihilated or eradicated; the patient literally was driven out of that part of the mind and brain.

Several years later, after having remained free from mental disorder, Regina gave birth to her first child. Proud of this accomplishment, she naturally wanted to share this with her mother. When the baby was six months old, she reestablished contact—only to have a recurrence of her acute illness.

This time when she refused medication it could not be given—at least not without lengthy court proceedings that might not succeed. Valuable time was lost and as a result she moved deeply into the psychosis. In her psychotic state, her infant mind "remembered" the tough fight with the first therapist and she sought the help of another doctor. She decided against medication, she reestablished the relationship with her original family and she never fully recovered.

Not only did the new regulation prevent an immediate recovery, but it resulted in a permanent illness that cost vast sums of money—which could have been used elsewhere in the health care system. Patients rights worked against her recovery and against the wishes of her adult mind.

Over the last two decades, countless lives have been lost and families have been destroyed as patients have been allowed to slip into permanent oblivion because of legislation *for* the patient.

The patient is one or two years old mentally and cannot determine what is in his or her best interest. If a small child needs to see a dentist, the parent takes the child whether the child wants to go or not. The patient needs to be protected and deserves kind and humane treatment, but treatment cannot be guided or directed by an irrational one year old brain. It is difficult enough for a skilled professional to bring about a recovery. There are not enough funds available to try to let the patient direct treatment.

It is still possible, through commitment proceedings, to hospital-ize a mental patient who is a danger to the self or others, or who can-not care for the self. With alcohol dependence the problem is much worse. The patient is allowed to commit suicide by drinking.

If the patient is alcohol dependent and is causing great harm to himself, this, too, is a form of insanity, a return to the infant on a bottle mind and brain, and it should be treated as such.

Instead of deciding that "he" has a right to drink as much as he wants, it should be realized that the "he" is one year old and cannot do otherwise. The person who is alcohol dependent must be forced to abstain long enough at least for the adult mind to resurface and make the decision. Brain atrophy and the corresponding signs of mild dementia reverse after six months, and therefore periodically a six month abstinence should be enforced—to give the adult mind and brain an opportunity to decide.

Alcohol and drug dependent individuals who have infants, tod-dlers or small children should be restricted even further. Young chil-dren or infants suffer enormously as a result of drug or alcohol dependent parents, and the damage is enduring. Once the diagnosis of substance dependence is made, and the person has young chil-dren, the process should be stopped. The parent should be given dai-ly testing or mandatory halfway house or hospitalization—and accompanied by the infant/toddler. The suffering and the damage to the child is so great that mandatory confinement should be enforced. Weeks or months should not be allowed to pass by. Seventy-two hours is ample time for definitive action.

Insanity Defense:

"Did he know what he was doing?" Which *he*?? The adult or the in-fant?

"Did he know what he was doing was wrong?" Which he??

"If he could drive a car or invest in the stock market, he must have known what he was doing." But which he was in charge and direct-ing the actions? When the infant is in charge, it can utilize some of the automatic functions of the adult.

"Was he functioning under diminished capacity?" This question indicates a more sophisticated level of understanding. The adult "he" was not present in full density—somewhat like a dot matrix newspaper photograph with every second dot missing. The question should be: "Where is the preponderance? In the adult mind and brain or in that of the infant?"

"How do you really tell which mind the person predominantly was using?" By the realities experienced at the time, by the bizarre behavior that correlates with the age at the time of the original trauma, by the dream like recall afterward, and by the inability of the adult mind to reconcile the actions of the infant mind—because they are incongruous with the morals and standards of the adult mind—once recovery has taken place.

In summary, the new understanding of serious emotional disorder—as explained in this text—calls for changes in mental health regulations pertaining to psychotic, suicidal, and drug and alcohol dependent individuals. Substance dependent parents in particular need external control for protection of the young, and the insanity defense has to decipher which "he" predominates and is in charge.

——21——

Peer Review and Regulations Governing Compensation

As with the section on treatment, the authors omit lengthy discussions of concepts described elsewhere and present only the unique views and perceptions that may have escaped the scrutiny and thoughts of others before us.

A trend is sweeping the field of medicine and is changing the way physicians practice. The trend is called health care reform, and includes managed health care, HMOs, governmental innovations and countless more. The notion is that the consumer will save lots of money. The results are contrary to expectations, however; costs continue to escalate as the art of medicine changes to the business of medicine and physicians fight to survive.

Formerly in the USSR, a job required three people, one to do the work and two to watch. While this failed miserably behind the Iron Curtain, it is pursued with great diligence here in western health care systems.

Instead of one person attending to the care of the patient, we have the physician, the hospital utilization review committee, and the insurance carrier, all deciding on the treatment the patient is to receive. Thus, the health care dollar is divided by three.

Now the physician is about to treat the patient, but he must spend equal time satisfying the hospital utilization review committee and

187

equal time attending to the needs of the insurance carrier by careful documentation in the chart. Divide by three again.

Fees in some instances have been reduced to the level of the Russian laborers, who regularly quipped: "They pretend to pay us and we pretend to work." Divide by three again.

Ultimately the physician is nicked by the insurance carrier that contends he failed to document treatment or necessity, and payment is denied. The physician is angered and tries to find a legal way to compensate for the difference. Divide by three again.

Insurance carriers and health maintenance organizations desperately race to plug loopholes while the ingenuity of the physician finds still more. He purchases a scanner, opens a biofeedback lab, or begins administering routine psychological tests. Divide by three again.

The physician has worked hard to achieve his status and his efforts deserve a just reward. If the health care system is to succeed, the physician must feel that compensation is commensurate with effort.

The caring, the dedication, the sincere efforts to help one's fellow man, are a part of love, which is the driving force behind the art of medicine. Making health care into an adversarial relationship, stirs needs and animosity, and robs the physician and the patient of the unique force that serves as the basis for recovery.

Business focuses on the bottom line: get as much as you can for as little as you can. This principle serves not the art of medicine, and it runs counter to the healing process.

In the field of psychiatry the efforts to control fees are based on time spent with the patient, since it is costly and time consuming to demonstrate psychological change. Thus, a skilled psychiatrist with psychoanalytic training is compensated only as much as a psychologist with no medical school, residency or psychoanalytic training. This system does not reward training or excellence, but it is enforceable because the highly skilled professionals comprise a small minority.

If this principle were applied to concerts, soloists would be docked for not holding a note the prescribed time and Yehudi Menuin could not charge more than a recent Julliard graduate. In sports, a Babe Ruth would receive the salary of a first year rookie, and in the auto industry, all cars weighing two tons and having four tires would cost $8,000.

Since this principle does not promote excellence in music, sports or industry, it is not likely to promote excellence in medicine.

Medicare regulations governing payment to psychiatrists are

stringent, as funds are scarce. In Pennsylvania, if one charges a dollar more than allowed, there is a $2,000 fine with a $5,000 fine the next time. If one charges a dollar less, it is labeled Medicare fraud. Payment is reduced further through mathematics. In psychiatry, the hourly allowance is approximately one-half to one-third of one's fee, and Medicare pays 50 percent of that. The 50 percent is referred to as 80 percent of 62 1/2 percent, which allows supplemental insurance carriers to advertise and sell policies that pay "the other 20 percent." Unfortunately, 20 percent of 62 1/2 percent is only 12 1/2 percent, which leaves another 37 1/2 percent unprotected. The doctor may feel threatened, deceived, tricked, forced to study regulations and to fill out forms—while the full allowable amount scarcely pays for office staff and expenses.

As more loopholes successively are found and then plugged, the noose tightens, the physician strangles, and his care and dedication become a fight for survival. The love disappears and with it the art. Before Leonardo da Vinci could paint the face of Jesus in The Last Supper, he had to visit his worst enemy to forgive and make amends. Hatred prevented him from capturing loving kindness in his art.

HMOs would plug all loopholes with capitation, but this innovation rewards the physician for not treating, and the patients suffer without care. The physician is paid the same to treat 20,000 patients, whether he sees any of them or not. Obviously, incentives to ignore health care problems are not a solution to health care needs.

In summary, the business solutions have been to squeeze either the doctor or the patient or both. We have seen that squeezing the doctor cannot solve the problems of health care reform because it stirs animosity, reduces the art of medicine and results in an unwilling caregiver. Squeezing the patient by disregarding the patient's needs hurts the patient and is counter to the Hippocratic oath. These innovations have failed.

Prior to health care reform, the physician simply did what he could to get the patient well, and charged his fee or whatever the patient could afford. This was a luxury. Now he must focus on regulations, complex documentation and filling out forms; he must contend with threats, fines, penalties and denial of payment for treatment rendered—any part of which can cause him to lose the spirit of helping the patient.

The large question is: How can the health care system return to the time when the physician's only concern was getting the patient well, with no incentive to undertreat the patient—such as created by

HMOs, and no tendency to overtreat—as brought about by carte blanche policies?

The answer may be simple, and could begin with self-insured companies. Suppose a physician were paid a high hourly wage, to treat a set number of patients, with the provision that as soon as he finishes treating one patient, that patient is replaced with another. By this means, there is no reason to undertreat the patient—as with HMOs—and there is no reason to overtreat the patient. This eliminates the need for managed health care. No more peer reviews, no more independent medical evaluations, no more documentation of necessity of treatment, no more rehabilitation nurses inspecting to see that the doctor is doing his job correctly. The physician gives the patient exactly what the physician thinks the patient needs, no more, no less. And then he goes on to help the next patient.

This chapter has been added as a second addendum to the Treatment Section of the text because movements in health care reform are impacting severely on treatment and quality of care, and because rising health care costs have prevented many patients from receiving treatment they desperately need.

APPENDIX

Appendix

Diagram "A"

Anxiety Disorders

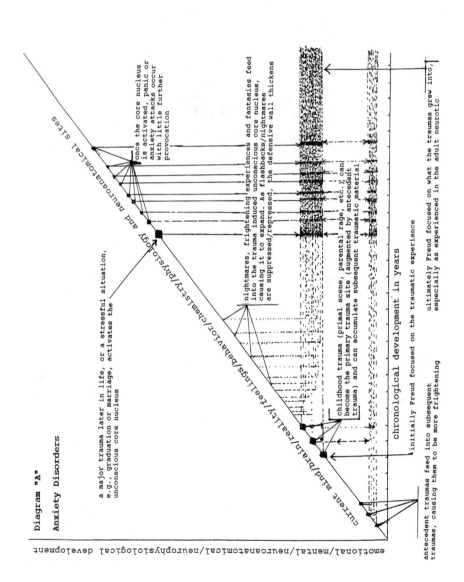

a major trauma later in life, or a stressful situation,
e.g., graduation or marriage, activates the
unconscious core nucleus

once the core nucleus
is activated, panic or
anxiety attacks occur
with little further
provocation

nightmares, frightening experiences and fantasies feed
into the trauma induced unconscious core nucleus,
causing it to expand. As flashbacks/nightmares
are suppressed/repressed, the defensive wall thickens

childhood trauma (primal scene, parental rage, etc.) can
become the primary trauma site (augmented by antecedent
trauma) and can accumulate subsequent traumatic material

chronological development in years

initially Freud focused on the traumatic experience

antecedent traumas feed into subsequent
traumas, causing them to be more frightening

ultimately Freud focused on what the traumas grew into,
especially as experienced in the adult neurotic

emotional/mental/neuroanatomical/neurophysiological development

current mind/brain/reality/feelings/behavior/chemistry/physiology and neuroanatomical sites

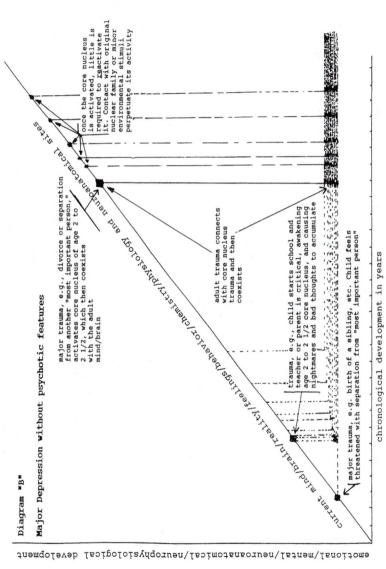

Diagram "B"

Major Depression without psychotic features

chronological development in years

emotional/mental/neuroanatomical/neurophysiological development

current mind/brain/reality/feelings/behavior/chemistry/physiology and neuroanatomical sites

major trauma, e.g., divorce or separation from another "most important person," activates core nucleus of age 2 to 2 1/2, which then coexists with the adult mind/brain

once the core nucleus is activated, little is required to reactivate it. Contact with original nuclear family or minor environmental stimuli perpetuate its activity

adult trauma connects with core nucleus trauma and then coexists

trauma, e.g., child starts school and teacher or parent is critical, awakening age 2 to 2 1/2 core nucleus, and causing nightmares and bad thoughts to accumulate

major trauma, e.g. birth of a sibling, etc. Child feels threatened with separation from "most important person"

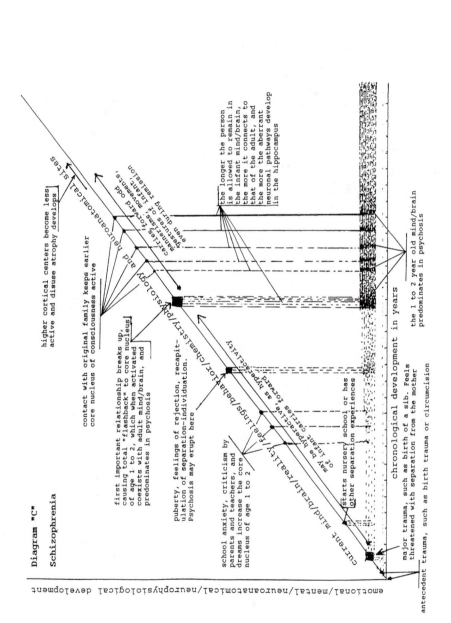

Diagram "C"

Schizophrenia

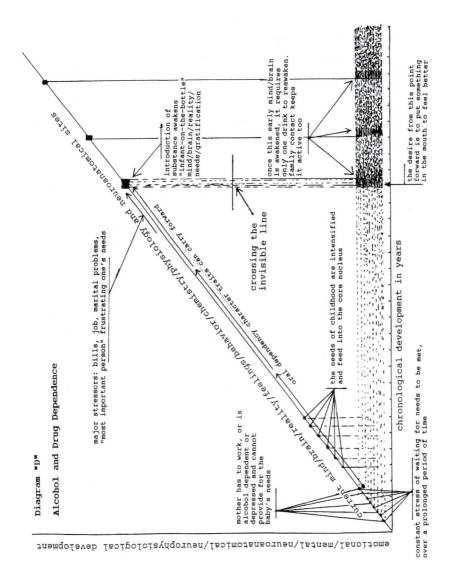

Diagram "D"

Alcohol and Drug Dependence

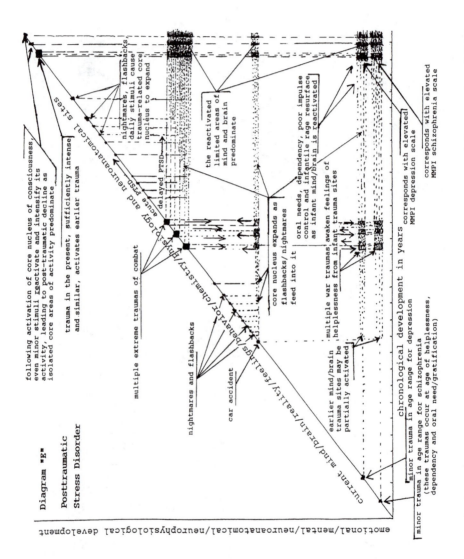

Diagram "E"

Posttraumatic
Stress Disorder

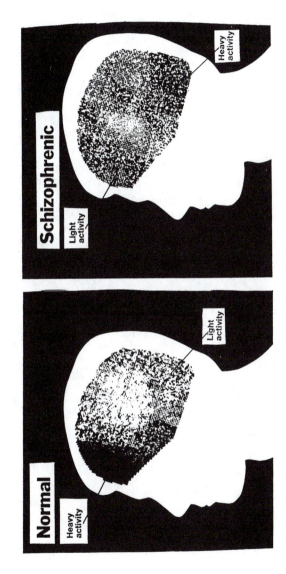

Diagram "F"

PET Scan Composites from NIMH

Bibliography

American Psychiatric Association. (1980). *Diagnostic and Statistical Manual of Mental Disorders* (third edition), Washington, D.C. p. 216.

American Psychiatric Association (1987). *Diagnostic and Statistical Manual of Mental Disorders* (third edition, revised), Washington, D.C.

American Psychiatric Association (1994). *Diagnostic and Statistical Manual of Mental Disorders (DSM-IV)*, Washington, D.C.

Andreason, N.C. (1983). *The Scale for the Assessment of Negative Symptoms (SANS)*. Monograph. University of Iowa, Iowa City, Iowa.

Andreason, N.C. (1984). *The Scale for the Assessment of Positive Symptoms (SAPS)*. Monograph. University of Iowa, Iowa City, Iowa.

Andreason N.C., Nasralla H.A., Dunn V.D., et al. (1986). Structural abnormalities in the frontal system in schizophrenia: a magnetic resonance imaging study. *Arch. Gen. Psychiatry*, 43: 136–144.

Andreason, N.C., Flaum, M., Swayze, V.W., Tyrrell, G., and Arndt, S. (1990). Positive and negative symptoms in schizophrenia. *Arch. Gen. Psychiatry*, 47: 615–621.

Andreason, N.C., Flaum, M. (1991a). Schizophrenia: the characteristic symptoms. *Schizophrenia Bulletin*. 17: No. 1, 27–49.

Andreason, N.C. and Flaum, M. (1991b). Diagnostic criteria for schizophrenia and related disorders: options for DSM-IV. *Schizophrenia Bulletin*. 17: No. 1, 133–142.

Andreason, N.C. & Flaum, M. (1991c). Appendix: Five criteria sets for DSM-IV field trials of schizophrenia and related disorders. *Schizophrenia Bulletin*. 17: No. 1, 143–156.

Andreason, N.C., Gupta, S., Flashman, L.A., Flaum, M.A., Nopoulos, P.C., O'Leary, D.S. (1994). Is the Neuropsychological Deficit in Schizophrenia Progressive? APA Meetings, May, 1994.

Angelones, A. (1990). Diagnosis of Personality disorders. APA Meeting, May 1990, New York.

Arnold, S.E. Franz, B., Gur, R.C., Gur, R.E., Trojanowski, J.Q. (1994). Neuronal Morphometric Studies of the Hippocampal Formation in Schizophrenia. APA Meetings, May, 1994, Philadelphia.

Atkenson, B.M., Calhoun, K.S., Resick, P.A., and Ellis, E.M. (1982). Victims of rape: Repeated assessment of depressive symptoms. *J. Consult. Clin. Psychol.* 50: 96–102.

Bark, N.M., DaSilva, D., Barros-Beck, J., Lindenmayer, S. (1994). Soft Neurological Signs and Dimensions of Schizophrenia. APA Meetings, May, 1994, Philadelphia.

Barr, C.E., Mednick, S.A., Munk-Jorgensen, P. (1990). Exposure to Influenza Epidemics During Gestation and Adult Schizophrenia. *Archives of General Psychiatry,* September 1990, 47: 869–874.

Barta, P.E., Pearlson, G.D., Powers, R.E., Richard, S.S. & Tune, L.E. (1990) *Am. J. Psychiatry,* 147: 1457–1462.

Baxter, L. (1994). PET Imaging in OCD and Depression. AMA Meetings, May, 1994, Philadelphia.

Beebe, G.W. (1975). Follow-up studies of World War II and Korean War prisoners. *Am. J. Epidemiol.* 101: 400–402.

Bellak, L., Hurvich, M., Gediman, H. (1973). *Ego Functions in Schizophrenics, Neurotics, and Normals.* John Wiley & Sons. New York.

Bettelheim, B. (1967). *The Empty Fortress: Infantile Autism and the Birth of Self.* Collier MacMillan Ltd. London. 484 pgs. The autistic anlage, p. 39–47; The right side of time, p. 47–57; Extreme situations, p. 63–68; In lieu of evidence, p. 351–366; Feral or autistic, p. 367–372.

Bettelheim, B. (1969). *The Children of the Dream: Infancy and Early Childhood.* Collier MacMillan Ltd. London. 363 pgs. Desertion, p. 92; The impermanent adult, p. 100; Autonomy, shame, doubt, p. 307.

Bleuler, E., Zinkin, J. (1950). *Dementia Praecox of the group of Schizophrenias.* International Universities Press. New York, N.Y.

Boffey, P.M. (1986). Schizophrenia. *New York Times,* March 16, 17, 18, 19, 1986.

Borus, J.F. (1973). Reentry: I. Adjustment issues facing the Vietnam returnee. *Arch. Gen. Psychiatry* 28: 501–506.

Bowlby, J. (1969). *Attachment and Loss, Volume 1, Attachment,* Basic Books, New York.

Bowlby, J. (1973). *Attachment and Loss, Volume 2, Separation,* Basic Books, New York.

Bowlby, J. (1984). Violence in the family as a disorder of the attachment and caregiving systems. *Am. J. Psychoanal.* 44: 9–27.

Breier, A.F. (1994). Dopamine, Stress & Schizophrenia. APA Meeting, May, 1994, Philadelphia.

Breier, A., Kelso, J., Kirwin, P., Beller, S., Wolkowitz, O., & Pickar, D. (1988). Early Parental Loss & Development of Adult Psychopathology. *Archives of General Psychiatry,* 45: 987–993.

Brett, E.A., and Ostroff, R. (1985). Imagery and post-traumatic stress disorder: An overview. *Am. J. Psychiat.* 142: 417–424.

Brown, G.L., Ebert, M.H., and Goyer, P. (1982). Aggression, suicide and sero-tonin. *Am. J. Psychiat.* 134: 741–745.

Brown, G.W. (1966). *Schizophrenia and Social Care: Comparative Follow-up Study 339 Schizophrenic Patients.* Maudsley Monograph, Oxford University Press, London, New York. 232 pps.

Brown, G.W., Wing, J.K. (1970). *Institutionalism and Schizophrenia: Study of Three Mental Hospitals,* 1960–1968.

University Press, Cambridge.

Brown, R., Colter, N., Corsellis, J.A.N., et al. (1986). Post-mortem evidence of structural changes in schizophrenia. *Arch Gen Psychiatry,* 43: 35–42.

Bunney, W.E., and Garland, B.L. (1984). Lithium and its possible mode of ac-tion. In Post, R.M., and Ballenger, J.C. (eds.), *Neurobiology of Mood Disor-ders,* Williams and Wilkins, Baltimore, pp. 731–743.

Burgess, A.W., and Holstrom, E. (1979). Adaptive strategies in recovery from rape. *Am. J. Psychiat.* 136: 1278–1282.

Burlingham, D. Empathy Between Infant and Mother. *J. Am. Psychoanalytic Association.* XV: 764–780.

Burman, B., Mednick, S.A., Machón, R.A., Parnas, J. & Schulsinger, F. (1987). Children at high risk for schizophrenia: Parent and offspring percep-tions of family relationships. *J. of Abnormal Psychology,* 1987, vol. 96, No. 4, 364–366.

Butler, P.D., Susser, E.s., Brown, A.s., Kaufman, C.A., Gorman, J.M. (1994). Malnutrition and Schizophrenia: Preclinical Studies, APA Meeting, May, 1994, Philadelphia.

Cancro, R. (1993). Schizophrenia Lecture. NYU/Bellevue Hospital Center Psychiatry Board Review, Feb. 26, 1993, NYC.

Cannon, T.D., Mednick, S.A., Parnas, J., Schulsinger, F., Praestholm, J., Vester-gaurd, A. (1993). Developmental brain abnormalities in the offspring of schizophrenic mothers. *Arch. Gen Psychiatry.* 50: 551–564, July, 1993.

Carlen, P.L., Penn, Sornazzani, Bennett, Wilkenson and Wortzman (1986). Computerized tomographic assessment of alcoholic brain damage and potential for reversibility. *J. of Alcoholism, Clinical and Experimental Re-search,* Volume 10, no. 3, pp. 226–232.

Center for Policy Research (1981). *Legacies of Vietnam: Comparative Adjustment of Veterans and Their Peers,* New York.

Cicchetti, D. (1984). The emergence of developmental psychopathology. *Child Dev.* 55: 1–7.

Coe, C.L., Mendoza, S.P., and Smotherman, W.P. (1978). Mother-infant at-tachment in the squirrel monkey: Adrenal responses to separation. *Be-hav. Biol.* 22: 256–263.

Crow, T.J. (1983). Is schizophrenia an infectious disease? *Lancit,* 1983; 1:173–175

Crow, T.J. (1990). Brain Structure in Psychosis and the Descent of Man. APA meeting, May 1990, New York.

Crow, T.J. (1994). The Death and the Replacement of the Kraepelinian Binary System. APA Meetings, May, 1994.

Crow, T.J., Done, D.J. (1992). Prenatal exposure to influenza does not cause schizophrenia. *Br. J. Psychiatry,* 1992; 161: 390–393.

Darwin, C. (1975). *On the Origin of the Species:* A Facsimile of the First [1859] Edition. Harvard University Press, Boston.

Davidson, G.E. (1985). Letter to Members of the American Society for Adolescent Psychiatry. Élan One Corp., Poland Spring, Maine.

Davidson, L.M., and Baum, A. (1986). Chronic stress and post-traumatic stress disorders. *J. Consult. Clin. Psychol.* 54: 303–308.

DeFazio, V. (1978). Dynamic perspectives on the nature and effects of combat stress. In Figley, C.R. (ed.), *Stress Disorders among Vietnam Veterans: Theory, Research, and Treatment Implications,* Brunner/Mazel, New York.

DeLisi, L.E. (1994). Can Brain Morphology Distinguish Genetic Subtypes? APA Meetings, May, 1994, Philadelphia.

Dewan, M.J., Masand, P., Thomas, F.D., Tanguary, J., Szeverenaji, N., Lynch, M. (1994). Correlates of SPECT Findings in Schizoprhenia. APA Meetings, May, 1994, Philadelphia.

Doman, G. (1974). *What to do About Your Brain Injured Child.* 1982 edition. The Better Baby Press, with Doubleday & Co. 291 pgs.

Doman, G. (1984). *How to Give Your Baby Encyclopedic Knowledge.* The Better Baby Press. Philadelphia. 302 pgs.

Doyle, J.S., and Bauer, S.K. (1989). Post-traumatic stress disorder in Children: Its identification and treatment in a residential setting for emotionally disturbed youth. *Journal of Traumatic Stress,* Vol. 2, No. 3, pp. 275–288

Dykes, K.L., Mednick, S.A., Machón, R.A., Praestholm, J., & Parnas, J. (1992). Adult third ventricle width and infant behavioral arousal in groups at high risk and low risk for schizophrenia. *Schizophrenia Research,* 7: 13–18, 192.

Emde, R.N. (1982). *The Development of Attachment and Affiliative Systems,* Plenum Press, New York.

Emery, P., and Smith, J. (1987). *The Treatment of Post-Traumatic Stress Disorder Based on Ten Propositions.*

Erikson, E.H. (1950). *Childhood and Society.* W.W. Norton & Co., New York, pp. 67–76, 219–234.

Eth, S., and Pynoos, R. (1985). *Post-traumatic Stress Disorder in Children,* American Psychiatric Press, Washington, D.C.

Eth, S., and Pynoos, R.S. (1985). Developmental perspective on psychic trauma in childhood. In Figley, C. (ed.), *Trauma and Its Wake,* Brunner/Mazel, New York, pp. 36–52.

Figley, C.R. (ed.). (1978). *Stress Disorders among Vietnam Veterans,* Brunner/Mazel, New York.

Figley, C.R. (1985). *Trauma & its Wake.* Vol 1. Brunner/Mazel, New York.

Frecksa, E., Greenberg, L., Sparks, J., Piscani, K. (1994). Selective Attention and Intention in Schizophrenia. APA Meeting, May, 1994, Philadelphia.

Freud, A. (1953). Some remarks on infant observation. *Psychoanalytic Study of the Child.* Vol. VIII. International Universities Press, New York, pp. 9–19.

Freud, A. (1954). Psychoanalysis and education. *Psychoanalytic Study of the Child*. Vol. IX. International Universities Press, New York, pp. 9–15.

Freud, A., and Bowlby, J. (1960) Grief and mourning in infancy and early childhood. *Psychoanalytic Study of the Child*, 15: 9–52.

Freud, A. (1963). The concept of developmental lines. *Psychoanalytic Study of the Child*, 18: 245–265.

Freud, S. (1894). The neuro-psychoses of defense. *Complete Psychological Works*, Standard Ed. Vo. 2. Translated and edited by Strachey J. London, Hogarth Press, 1954.

Freud, S. (1926). *The Problem of Anxiety*, Norton, New York.

Freud, S. (1958). *Remembering, Repeating, and Working Through (1914). Standard Edition of the Complete Psychological Works*, Vol. 12, Hogarth Press, London, pp. 147–156.

Freud, S. (1959). *Beyond the Pleasure Principle (1920). Standard Edition of the Complete Psychological Works*, Vol. 18, Hogarth Press, London, pp. 7–64.

Freud, S. (1961). The Ego and the Id (1923). *Standard Edition of the Complete Psychological Works*, Vol. 19, Hogarth Press, London.

Gampel, Y. (1988). Facing war, murder, torture and death in latency. *Psychoana. Rev.* 75.

Gampel, Y. (1989). I was a Holocaust child. In Wilson, A. (ed.), *The Holocaust Survivor and the Family*, In press.

Garfinkel, B. (1992). Child and adolescent psychiatry, Part I. *Psychiatric Times'* Intensive Review of Psychiatry and Neurology. Oct. 12–17, 1992.

Gil, T., Calev, A., Greenberg, D., Kugelmass, S., and Lerer, B. (1990). Cognitive functioning in post-traumatic stress disorder. *Journal of Traumatic Stress*, Vol. 3, No. 1, p. 29.

Goldman-Rakic, P.S. (1994). The Prefrontal Cortex and Working Memory. APA Meetings, May, 1994, Philadelphia.

Gordon, K.H. (1987) Psychiatric care for children with spinal injuries. *Pennsylvania Medicine*. 90: 60, 62. PA Med. Society, Leymoyne, PA, Sept., 1987.

Gordon, K.H., Rosenfeld, F. (1987). Prevention of symbiotic regression among high spinal cord injured adolescent boys and their mothers. *J. of Preventive Psychiatry*. Vol. 3, No. 4, 1987.

Green, B.L., Lindy, J.D., and Grace, M.C. (1985). Post-traumatic stress disorder: Toward DSM-IV. *J. Nerv. Ment. Dis.* 173: 406–411.

Green, B.L., Wilson, J.P., and Lindy, J.D. (1985). Conceptualizing PTSD: A psychosocial framework. In Figley, C.R. (ed.), *Trauma and Its Wake*, Brunner/Mazel, New York, pp. 53–69.

Grof, S. (1985). *Beyond the Brain: Birth, Death & Transcendence in Psychotherapy*. State University of New York Press. 466 pps., p. 307–315.

Gur, R.C., Gur, R.E., Mozley, L.H., Mozley, P.D., Shtasel, D.L., Alavi, A. (1994) Correlations Between Topography of Resting Metabolism and Clinical Presentation in Schizophrenia. APA Meetings, May, 1994, Philadelphia.

Gur, R.E., Gur, R.C., Shtasel, D.L., Gallacher, F., Turetsky, B. (1994). Brain Function in First Episode Schizophrenia. APA Meetings, May, 1994, Philadelphia.

Hagan, T. (1987). A retrospective search for the etiology of drug abuse: A background comparison of a drug addicted population of women and a control group of non-addicted women. *National Institute on Drug Abuse Monograph Series*, number 81, p. 254–261.

Harlow, H.F., and Woolsey, C.N. (1958). *Biological and Biochemical Bases of Behavior.* Halstead Press, pps. 355–357, 425–467.

Harlow, H.F, and Schrier, A.M. (1965). *Behavior of Non-human Primates* (2 vols.), New York Academic Press.

Harlow, H.F. (1971). *Learning to Love.* Albion Publishing Co., San Francisco. 122 pps.

Harlow, H.F. (1979). *The Human Model: Primate Perspectives.* Halstead Press.

Helzer, J.E., Robins, L.N., and McEvoy, L. (1987). Post-traumatic stress disorder in the general population. *N. Engl. J. Med.* 26: 1630–1634.

Hendin, H., Pollinger, Haas A., and Singer, P. (1983). The influence of precombat personality on post-traumatic stress disorders. *Comp. Psychiat.* 24: 530–534.

Hoffman, W.F., Burry, M.T., Keepers, G.A., Casey, D.E. (1991). Unexpected intracerebral pathology in older schizophrenic patients. *Am. J. Psychiatry.* 148:3, pp. 390–391.

Hokama, H., Shenton, M.E., Kikinis, R., Wible, C.G., Jolesz, F.A., McCarley, R.W. (1994). Three-Dimensional Brain Atlas From Magnetic Resonance Data. APA Meetings, May, 1994, Philadelphia.

Holmes, T. (1967). The Holmes and Rahe social readjustment rating scale. *J. Psychometr. Res.* 11: 213–218.

Holzman, P.S. (1994). Spatial Working Memory and Eye Movement Deficits. APA Meetings, May, 1994, Philadelphia.

Horowitz, M. (1976). *Stress Response Syndromes*, Aronson, New York.

Horowitz, M.J. (1977). Phase oriented treatment of stress response syndrome. *Am. J. Psychother.* 31: 38–42.

Hough, R.L., Vega, W., Valle, R., Kolody, B., Griswald del Castillo, R., and Tarke, H. (1990). Mental health consequences of the San Ysidro McDonald's massacre: A community study. *Journal of Traumatic Stress*, Vol. 3, No. 1, p. 71.

Huttunen, M.O., Niskanen, P. (1978). Prenatal loss of father and psychiatric disorders. *Arch. Gen. Psychiatry,* 1978; 35: 429–431.

Hyman, I.A., Zelikoff, W., and Clarke J. (1988). Psychological and physical abuse in the schools: A paradigm for understanding post-traumatic stress disorder in children and youth. *Journal of Traumatic Stress*, Vol. 1, No. 2, p. 243.

Janet, P. (1886). Les actes inconscients et la mémoire pendant le somnambulisme. *Rev. Philos.* 25(I): 238–279.

Janet, P. (1893). L'Amnésie continue. *Rev. Gen. Sci.* 4: 167–179.

Janet, P. (1894). Histoire d'une idee fixe. *Rev. Philos.* 37: 121–168.

Janet, P. (1897). L'insomnie par idee fixe subconsciente. *Presse Med.* 5: 41–44.

Janet, P. (1903). *Les Obsessions et la Psychasthenie* (2 vol.), Alcan, Paris.

Janet, P. (1904). L'Amnesie et la dissociation des souvenirs par l'emotion. *J. Psychol.* 4: 417–453.

Janet, P. (1909). *Les Nevroses*, Flammarion, Paris.

Janet, P. (1919). Les medications psychologiques (3 volumes), Alcan, Paris.

Janet, P. (1973). *L'Automatisme Psychologique: Essay de Psychologie Experimentale sur les Formes Inferieures de l'Active Humaine*, Paris, Felix Alcan, 1889. Reprint: Société Pierre Janet/Payot, Paris, 1973.

Janis, I.L. (1965). Psychodynamic aspects of stress tolerance. In Klausner, S.A. (ed.), *The Quest for Self-Control*, Free Press, New York, pp. 215–246.

Johnson, M.H., and Holzman, P.S. (1979). *Assessing Schizophrenic Thinking*, Jossey-Bass, San Francisco.

Jones, P.B., Murray, R.M., Rodgers, B. (1994). Developmental Trajectories to Adult Schizophrenia. APA Meetings, May, 1994, Philadelphia.

Kaplan, H.I. & Sadock, B.J. (1994). *Synopsis of Psychiatry*, Seventh Edition. Williams & Wilkins.

Kardiner, A. (1941). *The Traumatic Neuroses of War. Psychosomatic Medicine Monograph II-III*, National Research Council, Washington, D.C.

Katan, C. (1990). Chronic Mental Illness. APA Meeting, May 1990, New York.

Kaufman, C.A., Weinberger, D.R., Stevens, J.R. et al. (1988). Intracerebral innoculation of experimental animals with brain tissue from patients with schizophrenia. *Arch. Gen. Psychiatry*, 1988; 45: 648–652.

Keane, T.M., and Kalupek, D.G. (1982). Imaginal flooding in the treatment of post-traumatic stress disorder. *J. Consult. Clin. Psychol.* 50: 138–140.

Kernberg, O. (1975). *Borderline Condition & Pathological Narcisism*. Jason Aronson, Inc. N.Y.

Kestenberg, J.S. (1982). A metapsychological assessment based on an analysis of a survivor's child. In Bergman, N.S., and Jucovy, M.E. (eds.), *Generations of the Holocaust*, Basic Books, New York.

Kestenberg, J.S. (1987). Imagining and remembering. Unpublished paper, Sands Point, New York.

Kestenberg, J.S., and Brenner, I. (1986). Children who survived the holocaust. *Int. J. Psychanal.* 67: 309–316.

Khan, M. (1983). The concept of cumulative trauma. *Psychoanal. Study Child* 18: 54–58.

Kilpatrick, D.G., Veronen, L.J., and Best, C.L. (1985). Factors predicting psychological distress among rape victims. In Figley, C.R. (ed.), *Trauma and Its Wake*, Brunner/Mazel, New York, pp. 113–141.

Kinzie, J.D. (1989). Therapeutic approaches to traumatized Cambodian refugees. *Journal of Traumatic Stress*, Vol. 2, No. 1.

Kinzie, J.D., and Boehnlein, J.J. (1989). Post-traumatic psychosis among Cambodian refugees. *Journal of Traumatic Stress*, Vol. 2, No. 2.

Koegler, R.R., and Hicks, S.M. (1972). The destruction of a medical center by earthquake: Initial effects on patients and staff. *Calif. Med.* 116: 63–67.

Kolb, L. (1987). Neuropsychological hypothesis explaining post-traumatic stress disorder. *Am. J. Psychiat.* 144: 989–995.

Konner, M. (1982). Biological aspects of the mother-infant bond. In Emde, R.N., and Harmon, R.J. (eds.), *The Development of Attachment and Affiliative Systems*. Plenum, New York.

Kraemer, G.W., Ebert, M.H., Lake, C.R., and McKinney, G.W. (1984). Hypersensitivity to d-amphetamine several years after early social deprivation in rhesus monkeys. *Psychopharmacology* 82: 266–271.

Kraepelin, E., Barclay, R.M., Robertson, G.M. (1919). *Dementia Praecox and Paraphrenia*. E & S Livingstone. Edinburgh, Scotland.

Kris, E. (1956). The recovery of childhood memories. *Psychoanal. Study Child* 11: 54–58.

Krystal, H. (1968). *Massive Psychic Trauma*, International Universities Press, New York.

Krystal, H. (1984). Psychoanalytic views on human emotional damages. In van der Kolk, B. (ed.), *Post-traumatic Stress Disorder: Psychological and Biological Sequelae*, APA Press, Washington, D.C., pp. 1–28.

Krystal, J. (1978). Trauma and effects. *Psychoanal. Study Child* 33: 81–116.

Krystal, J.H., Larvelle, M., Abi-Darghaur, A. Seibyl, J.P., Karpor, L.P., Charney, D.S. (1994). Serotonin and Schizophrenia. APA Meetings, May, 1994, Philadelphia.

Lane, A., Kinsella, A., Murphy, P., Waddington, J.L., Larkin, C., O'Callaghn, E. (1994). Craniofacial Anomalies in Schizophrenia: Clues to the Timing of Developmental Disturbance. APA Meetings, May, 1994, Philadelphia.

Laudenslager, M., Capitano, J.P., and Reite, M. (1985). Possible effects of early separation on subsequent immune function in adult macaque monkeys. *Am. J. Psychiat.* 142: 862–864.

Lewin, B. (1946). Sleep, the mouth and the dream sequence. *Psychoanalytic Quarterly*, Volume 15, pp. 419–434.

Lewin, B. (1958). Dreams and the uses of regression. Monograph. Freud Anniversary Lecture Series of the New York Psychoanalytic Institute. International Universities Press. New York.

Lifton, R.J., and Olson, E. (1976). The human meaning of total disaster: The Buffalo Creek experience. *Psychiatry* 39: 1–18.

Lindemann, H. (1944). Symptomatology and management of acute grief. *Am. J. Psychiatry* 101: 141.

Lowen, A. (1958). *Physical Dynamics of Character Structure; Bodily Form and Movement in Analytic Therapy.* Grune and Stratton, New York, 358 pps.

Lowen, A. (1975). *Love and Orgasm.* Collier Books, New York, 319 pps.

Lyons, J.A., Gerardi, R.J., Wolfe, J., and Keane, T.M. (1988).Multidimensional assessment of combat-related PTSD: Phenomenological, psychometric, and psychophysiological considerations. *Journal of Traumatic Stress*, Vol. 1, No. 3., pp. 376–377.

MacLean, P.D. (1973). *A Triune Concept of the Brain and Behavior.* The Clarence M. Hicks Memorial Lectures 1969 for Ontario Mental Health Foundation, University of Toronto Press, 165 pps.

MacLean, P.D. (1985). Brain evolution relating to family, play and the separation call. *Arch. Gen. Psychiat.* 42: 505–417.

Mahler, M.S., and Gosliner, B.J. (1955). On symbiotic child psychosis, genetic, dynamic and restitutive aspects. *Psychoanalytic Study of the Child*, Vol. X. International Universities Press, New York. pp. 195–212.

Mahler, M.S., and Furer, M. (1968) *On Human Symbiosis and the Vicissitudes of Individuation* (2 vols.). International Universities Press, New York.

Mahler, M.S. (1979). *The Selected Papers of Margaret S. Mahler, M.D.* (2 vols.). V. Aronson Publisher, New York, 242 pps.

Malhorta, A.K., Su, T.P., Kammerer, W., Pickar, D., Breier, A.F. (1994). Glutamatergic Hypothesis of Schizophrenia. APA Meetings, May, 1994, Philadelphia.

Masterson, J.F. (1978). *New Perspectives on Psychotherapy of the Borderline Adult*; contributions by P.L. Givacchini, Ottoa F. Kernberg, James F. Masterson & Harold F. Searles. Brunner/ Mazel. N.Y.

Mathew, R.J., M.R.C. Psyche., and C. Leon Partain (1985). Midsagital sections of the cerebeallar vermis and fourth ventricle obtained with magnetic resonance imaging of schizophrenic patients. *Am. J. Psychiatry.* 142:8.

Mazor, A., Gampel, Y, Enright, R.D., and Orenstein, R. (1990). Holocaust survivors: Coping with post-traumatic memories in childhood and 40 years later. *Journal of Traumatic Stress*, Vol. 3, No. 1, p. 1.

McCarley, R.W., Shenton, M.E., Kikinis, R., Wible, C.G., Dengler, J., Jolesz, F.A. (1994). At Warp Speed: MRI Windows on the Brain and Behavior. APA Meetings, May, 1994, Philadelphia.

McCormick, R.A., Taber, J.I., and Kruedelbach, N. (1989). The relationship between attributional style and post-traumatic stress disorder in addicted patients. *Journal of Traumatic Stress*, Vol. 2, No. 4, p. 485.

McKenzie, C. (1981). Schizophrenia and the McKenzie Method. Audio Tape Cassettes. American Health Association. Box 345, Bala Cynwyd, PA.

McKenzie, C. & Wright, L.S. (1981). The Consciousness Movement, Silva Mind Control and the Mental Patient; Evaluation of 189 patients. *Voices: Journal of the American Academy of Psychotherapists*, Vol. 17, #1, pp. 56–64.

McKenzie, C. (1982). Programmed Dreams: A Breakthrough in Medical & Psychiatric Diagnosis & Treatment. American Health Association. Box 345, Bala Cynwyd, PA.

McKenzie, C. (1983) *Defining Love Energy; Combining Clinical Observations with Eastern Philosophy.* Lecture, International Primal Association, Philadelphia Spring Conference. Monograph, American Health Association, Box 345, Bala Cynwyd, PA.

McKenzie, C. (1984). *The Anatomy & Psychodynamics of Psychosis.* Lecture, International Congress in Madrid. Monograph, American Health Association. Box 345, Bala Cynwyd, PA.

McKenzie, C. (1986a). *Having Schizophrenia is Unnecessary.* Lecture Series at the Philadelphia County Medical Society.

McKenzie, C. (1986b). *A Correlation Between Early Infant Trauma and Serious Emotional Disorders.* Monograph, American Health Association, Box 345, Bala Cynwyd, PA.

McKenzie, C. (1992). Deciphering a schizophrenia cause. *Medical Tribune.* Vol. 33, Number 18.

McKenzie, C (1993a). *Neuropsychiatric Damages Assessments of 41 Victims of October 4, 1992 Boeing 747 El Al Airline Crash in Bijlmermeer, Holland.* American Health Association. Bala Cynwyd, PA. 150 pp.

McKenzie, C (1993b). *Neuropsychiatric Damages Assessments of 51 Victims of July 18, 1993 Sahsa Airline Crash in Managua, Nicaragua.* American Health Association. Bala Cynwyd, PA. 200 pp.

McKenzie, C. and Sullivan, R. (unpublished). *When the Baby Kills.*

Mednick, S.A., Machón, R.A., Huttunen, M.O., Bonett, D. (1988). Adult schizophrenia following prenatal exposure to an influenza epidemic. *Archives of General Psychiatry,* February, 1988, 45: 189–192.

Mednick, S.A., Parnas, J., & Schulsinger, F. (1987). *Schizophrenia Buletin.* Vol. 13, No. 3, pps. 485–495, 1987.

Meisner, W.N. (1977). Family process and psychosomatic disease. In Lipowski, Z.L., Lipsitt, O., and Witybrow, P. (eds.), *Psychosomatic Medicine,* Oxford Press, New York.

Mueller, T.I., Lavori, P.W., Keller, M.B., Schwartz, A., Warshaw, M.G., Hasin, D. (1994). Effect of Alcoholism on a Ten Year Course of Depression. APA Meetings, May, 1994, Philadelphia.

Murray, R.M, Jones, P.B., Walsh, C. (1994). Difference in Age of Onset and Brain Structure. APA Meetings, May, 1994, Philadelphia.

Museso, C., Young, A. (1974). *Consciousness and Reality.* Avon Books, New York.

Nasrallah, H.A., Ketterer, M., Sharma, S.K., Olson, S.C., Martin, R., Lynn, M.B. (1994). Decreased Hippocampal Volume Over Time in Schizophrenia: Evidence of Neurodegeneration. APA Meetings, May, 1994, Philadelphia.

Nelson, J. Craig (1992). Schizophrenia. *Psychiatric Times'* Intensive Review of Psychiatry and Neurology, October, 1992.

Nemeroff, C.B. (1993). The Psychoneuroendocrinology of Depression: Hypothalmic—Pituitary—Adrenal Axis Dysregulation. *Strecker Monograph Series XXX,* November, 1993, Institute of the Pennsylvania Hospital, Philadelphia.

Nemeroff, C.B. (1994). Neuropeptides and schizophrenia. APA Meeting, May, 1994, Philadelphia.

Nestor, P.G., Shenton, M.E., Wible, C.G., Kimble, M.O., Smith, L., McCarley, R.W. (1994). Schizophrenia: Neuropsychological and MRI Findings. APA Meetings, May, 1994, Philadelphia.

Niznikiewicz, M.A., O'Donnell, B.F., McCarley, R.W. (1994). Event Related Potential Indices of Language Problems in Schizophrenia. APA Meetings, May, 1994, Philadelphia.

O'Donnell, B.F., Faux, S.F., McCarley, R.W., Shenton, M.E., Kimble, M.O., Nestor, P.Q. (1994). Event Related Potential and MRI Evidence of Deterioration in Schizophrenia. APA Meetings, May, 1994, Philadelphia.

Pearce, J.C. (1977). *Magical Child*. E.P. Dutton, New York.

Pearce, J.C. (1985). *Magical Child Matures*. E.P. Dutton, New York. 235 pps.

Pearson, G.H.J. (1958). *Adolescence & The Conflict of Generations*. W.W. Norton & Co., Inc. New York. pp. 18–28; 144–158.

Pearlson, G.D., Kim, W.S., Kubos, K.L., et al. (1989). Ventricle-brain ration, computerized tomographic density and brain area in 50 schizophrenics. *Arch. Gen. Psychiatry.* 46: 690–697.

Pearlson, G.,D., Barta, P.E., Schlaepfer, T.E., Petty, R.G., Tien, A.Y., McGilchrist, I.K. (1994). Heteromodal Association Cortex in Schizophrenia. APA Meetings, May, 1994, Philadelphia.

Perkins, D.O., Gilmore, C.S. (1994). Fluctuating Derniatoglyphic Asymmetry, HLA Homozygosity and Schizophrenia. APA Meetings, May, 1994, Philadelphia.

Piaget, J. (1936). *The Origins of Intelligence in Children*. International Universities Press. New York, 1952.

Pynoos, R., and Eth, S. (1985). Developmental perspectives on psychic trauma. In Figley, C.R. (ed.), *Trauma and Its Wake*, Brunner/Mazel, New York, pp. 36–52

Pynoos, R.S., and Nader, K. (1988). Psychological first aid and treatment approach to children exposed to community violence: Research implications. *Journal of Traumatic Stress*, Vol. 1, No. 4, p. 461, 471.

Raifman, L.J. (1983). Problems of diagnosis and legal causation in courtroom use of post-traumatic stress disorder. *Behav. Sci. Law* 1(3): 115–130.

Rajecki, D.W., Lamb, M.E., and Obmascher, P. (1978). Toward a general theory of infantile attachment: A comparative review of aspects of the social bond. *Behav. Brain Sci.* 3: 417–464.

Raphael, B. (1977). The Granville train disaster: Psychological needs and their management. *Med. J. Austr.* 1: 303–305.

Reite, M., Short, R., and Seiler, C. (1981). Attachment, loss and depression. *J. Child Psychol. Psychiat.* 22: 141–169.

Rochlin, G. (1953). Loss and restitution. *Psychoanalytic Study of the Child*, Vol. VIII. International Universities Press, New York. pp. 288–309.

Rossi, A., Stratta, P., Mancini, F., Mattei, P., Cassachia, M. (1994). Amygdala—Anterior Hippocampus Shrinkage in Male Schizophenia: A Magnetic Resonance Controlled Study. APA Meetings, May, 1994, Philadelphia.

Roy, M., Crowe, R.R. (1994). Are Familial and Sporadic Subtypes of Schizophrenia Valid? APA Meetings, May, 1994, Philadelphia.

Russell, J.M., Vitlanueva-Mey, J., Early, T.S., Martin, J.L. (1994). Temporal Lobe Asymmetries in Functional Psychosis. APA Meetings, May, 1994, Philadelphia.

Samuel, T. (1990). Vietnam's delayed hit. *Philadelphia Inquirer*, May 28, 1990, p. E-1.

Schmale, A. (1958). The relationship of separation and depression to disease. *Psychosom. Med.* 20: 259.

Schneck, H. (1986). Schizophrenic focus changes to dramatic changes in the brain. *New York Times, Science Times.* March 18, 1986.

Schwartz, S.R., Africa, B. (1988). Schizophrenic Disorders. In: Goldman, H.H., ed. *Review of General Psychiatry.* Norwalk: Appleton & Lange; 1988.

Schwartz, Lee S. (1990). A biopsychosocial treatment approach to post-traumatic stress disorder. *Journal of Traumatic Stress*, Vol. 3, No. 2, p. 223.

Seligman, M. (1969). *Psychology Today.* June, 1962.

Sharron, A. (1988). Madness and temporality: Reviewing and reconsidering an old hypothesis of schizophrenia. *Studies in Symbolic Interaction*, Vol. 9, pp. 111–126.

Shedlack, K.J., Lee, G.R., Sakuna, M., Pepple, J.R., Hoff, A.L., DeLisi, L.E. (1994). Impaired Memory and Attention Associated with Abnormal Brain Morphology in Schizophrenia Multiplex Families. APA Meetings, May, 1994, Philadelphia.

Shenton, M.E., Nestor, P., O'Donnell, B., Wible, C.G., Kikinas, R., McCarley, R.W. (1994). The Superior Temporal Gyrus and Thought Disorder. APA Meetings, May, 1994, Philadelphia.

Silva, J. and Miele, P. (1977). *The Silva Mind Control Method.* Simon & Schuster, New York. 239 pps.

Silverstein, M.L., Silver, M., Harrow, M. (1994). Neuro-psychological Functions and Clinical OUtcome. APA Meetings, May, 1994, Philadelphia.

Sokoloff, L. (1994). Brain Local Functional Activity: Metabolic Mapping. APA Meetings, May, 1994, Philadelphia.

Spitz, R. (1945). Hospitalism: An inquiry into the genesis of psychiatric conditions in early childhood. *Psychoanalytic Study Child* 1: 53–74.

Spitz, R. (1983). Dialogues from infancy. *Selected Papers.* International Universities Press, New York.

Spitz, R.A., Cobliner, W.G. (1975). Emotional deficiency diseases of the infant. *The First Year of Life.* International Universities Press, pps. 267–300.

Spitzer, R.L., and Williams, J.B. (1985a). Proposed revisions in the DSM-III classification of anxiety disorders based on research and clinical experience. In Tuma, A.H., and Master, J.D. (eds.), *Anxiety and the Anxiety Disorders*, Hillsdale, N.J., Lawrence Erlbaum Associates, pp. 759–774.

Stains, L.R. (1987). Daycare: The Quiet Crisis. *Philadelphia Magazine*, September 1, 1987.

Stretch, R. (1985). Post-traumatic stress disorder among U.S. Army Reserve Vietnam and Vietnam-Era veterans. *J. Consult. Clin. Psychol.* 53: 935–936

Stretch, R. (1986a). Incidence and etiology of post-traumatic stress disorder among active duty Army personnel. *J. Appl. Social Psychol.* 16: 464–481.

Stretch, R. (1986b). Post-traumatic stress disorder among Vietnam and Vietnam-era veterans. In Figley, C.R. (ed.), *Trauma and Its Wake, Volume II: Traumatic Stress Theory, Research and Intervention*, Brunner/Mazel, New York, pp. 156–192.

Stretch, R.H. (1990). Post-traumatic stress disorder and the Canadian Vietnam veteran. *Journal of Traumatic Stress*, Vol. 3, No. 2, p. 248.

Suddath, R.L., Casanova, M.F., Goldberg, T.E., et al. (1989) Temporal lobe pathology in schizophrenia: a quantative resonance imaging study. *Am. J. Psychiatry*, 146: 464–472.

Suddath, R.L., Christison, G.W., Torrey, E.F., Casanova, M.F., and Weinberger, D.R. (1990). Anatomical abnormalities in the brains of monozygotic twins discordant for schizophrenia. *N. Engl. J. Med.* 322: 789–94.

Talbot, A. (1990). The importance of parallel process in debriefing crisis counselors. *Journal of Traumatic Stress*, Vol. 3, No. 2, p. 269.

Tart, C. (1969). *Altered States of Consciousness*. John Wiley & Sons, New York.

Tausk, V. (1933). The origin of the "influencing machine" in schizophrenia. *Psa. Quarterly.* II: 519–556, reproduced from *Int'l. Zeitschrift für Psychoanalys.* (1919).

Tennes, K. (1982). The role of hormones in mother-infant transactions. In Emde, R.N., and Harmon, R.J. (eds.), *The Development of Attachment and Affiliative Systems*, Plenum, New York, pp. 75–80.

Terr, L.C. (1994). Early Intervention for Childhood Trauma, or Else? APA Meetings, May, 1994, Philadelphia.

U.S. Dept. of Health and Human Services. (1988). *Vital Statistics of the United States, 1986.* Volume 1, Natality. National Center for Health Statistics. Hyattsville, MD. pp. 44–293.

van der Kolk, B.A., and Ducey, C.P. (1984). Clinical implications of the Rorschach in post-traumatic stress disorder. In van der Kolk, B.A. (ed.), *Post-Traumatic Stress Disorder: Psychological and Biological Sequelae*, American Psychiatric Press, Washington.

van der Kolk, B.A., and Ducey, C.P. (1989). The psychological processing of traumatic experience: Rorschach patterns in PTSD. *Journal of Traumatic Stress*, Vol. 2, No. 3, p. 265–267.

van der Kolk, B.A., Herman, J.L., and Perry, C. (1987). *Traumatic antecedents of borderline personality disorder*, Paper presented at the Fourth Annual Meeting of the Society for Traumatic Stress Studies, Baltimore.

van der Kolk, B.A. (1988). The trauma spectrum: The interaction of biological and social events in the genesis of the trauma response. *Journal of Traumatic Stress*, Vol. 1, No. 3, p. 277–279.

van der Kolk, B.A., Brown, P., and van der Hart, O. (1989). Pierre Janet on post-traumatic stress. *Journal of Traumatic Stress*, Vol. 2, No. 4, p. 365.

van der Ploeg, H.M., and Kleijn, W.C. (1989). Being held hostage in The Netherlands: A study of long-term aftereffects. *Journal of Traumatic Stress*, Vol. 2, No. 2, p. 154, 166.

van Kammen, D.P., Gurklis, J.A., Peters, J.L., Kelly, P.A., Yao, J.K. (1994). A Role of Norepinephrins in Schizophrenia. APA Meetings, May, 1994, Philadelphia.

Weinberger, D.R. (1994a). Neuroanatomical Perspectives on Schizophrenia. APA Meetings, May, 1994, Philadelphia.

Weinberger, D.R. (1994b). Insights from Neuroimaging about Schizophrenia. APA Meetings, May, 1994, Philadelphia.

Weinberger, D.R., Berman, K.F., Ostrem, J., Gold, J., Goldberg, T.E., Mattay, V.A. (1994). Functional Brain Imaging with PET Reconsidered. APA Meetings, May, 1994, Philadelphia.

Williams, J.S., and Siegel, J.P. (1989). Marital disruption and physical illness: The impact of divorce and spouse death on illness. *Journal of Traumatic Stress*, Vol. 2, No. 4, p. 555.

Wilson, J, and Walker, A. (1990). Toward an MMPI trauma profile. *Journal of Traumatic Stress*, Vol. 3, No. 1, pp. 151–168.

Wood, E., Paley, Sharon (1989). Balancing the Psychiatric Career and Motherhood. APA Meeting, May, 1989, San Francisco.

Wu, H., Munne, R., Bilder, R., Bogerts, B., Lieberman, J.A. (1994). Increased Inter-Putamen Distance—Brain Width Ratio in First Episode and Chronic Schizophrenic Patients. APA Meetings, May, 1994, Philadelphia.

Wyatt, R.J. (1994). Schizophrenia as a Limited Degenerative Brain Disorder. APA Meetings, May, 1994, Philadelphia.

Zelikoff, W. (1986). Evidence for a new diagnostic construct: Educator-induced post traumatic stress disorder. Unpublished manuscript, Temple University, Philadelphia.

Zill, N. (1985). Behavior and learning problems among adopted children: Findings from a U.S. national survey of child health. Child Trends, Inc., Washington, D.C.

Index